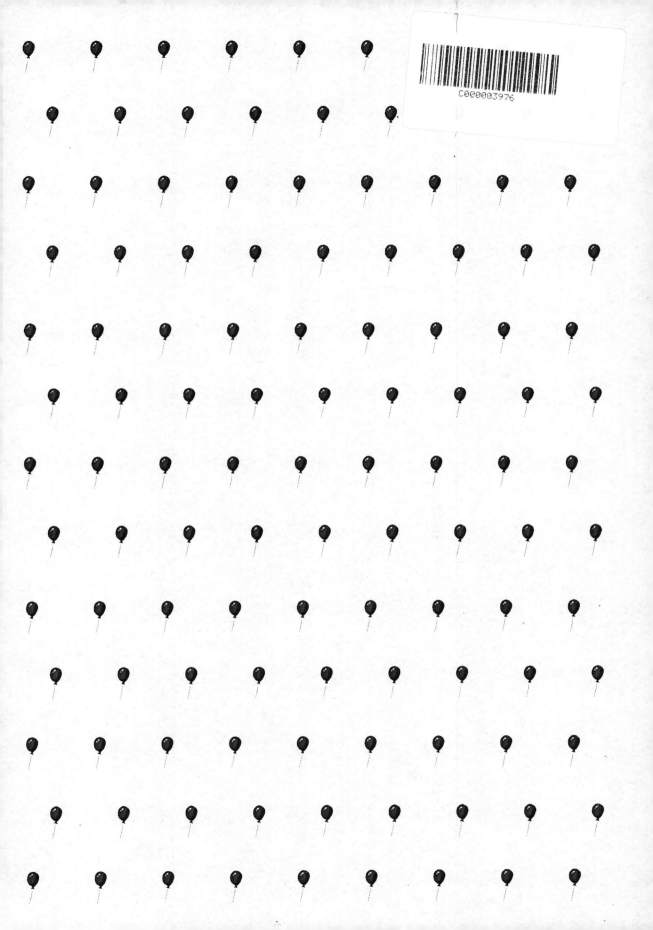

AUBRI TALLENT, ANDREI TALLENT
& FREDY BUSH

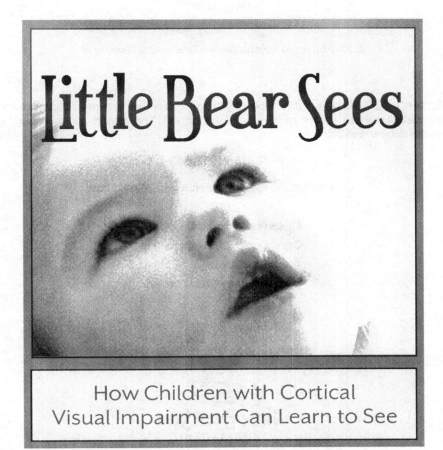

Little Bear Sees

How Children with Cortical
Visual Impairment Can Learn to See

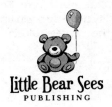

Little Bear Sees
PUBLISHING

Little Bear Sees:
How Children with Cortical Visual Impairment Can Learn to See

By
Aubri Tallent, Andrei Tallent
and
Fredy Bush

ISBN: 978-1-936214-82-2

Library of Congress Control Number: 2012936089

Cover Photo by Andrei Tallent
Cover Design by Nancy Cleary
Illustrations by Jason Nobriga
Logo design by 3200 Creative

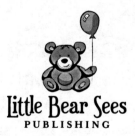

Little Bear Sees
PUBLISHING
Published by Little Bear Sees Publishing, a Wyatt-MacKenzie Imprint

Limits of Liability and Disclaimer of Warranty

The purpose of this book is to educate and inform. The authors and/or publisher and/or writer/editor shall have neither liability nor responsibility to anyone with respect to any loss or damage caused, or alleged to be caused, directly or indirectly by the information contained in this book.

Dedication

This book is lovingly dedicated to our Little Bear, Lukas Timothy Tallent. Without him, we would not have found our courage, our strength, our hope and our voices in advocating for children with CVI. We never expected to find ourselves on this journey, but we are so thankful to have Lukas in our lives and for all the beauty we have discovered along the way.

Table of Contents

Foreword By Christine Roman-Lantzy, Ph.D. ix

1 Little Bear Sees 1
 Meet Little Bear 1
 At the Beginning 3
 Fitting Puzzle Pieces Together for Little Bear 4
 Creating a Vision Routine 6
 Why We Wrote this Book 9
 "I Don't Believe It" Responses Are Good 10
 What You Will Learn 11

2 The Importance of Family and Bonding 13
 The Importance of Family 13
 The Importance of Bonding 14
 Follow the Child's Lead 16
 The Defining Moments 18
 Lukas' Grandmother's Inspiration 19
 Krista's Advocacy 20
 Kevin and Alicia's Emotional Roller Coaster 21
 Signs of the Blues and Depression 24

3 Cortical Visual Impairment 27
 What is Cortical Visual Impairment (CVI)? 27
 What Causes CVI? 29
 How Many Children Have CVI? 30
 Diagnosis 31
 Characteristics of CVI 32
 After the Diagnosis 35

4 Vision. . . the Gateway to the World? 37
 Visual Development 38
 How the Eyes and Brain Work Together 40
 Reception and Recognition 42
 Spatial Orientation 43
 Visual Reflexes 44
 Visual Fields 44
 Vision's Role in Learning 45
 Visual Pathways and Brain Injury 45

5 The Champines - A Diagnosis of CVI 51
 The Champines' First Months 51
 Getting a Diagnosis 53
 Learning How to Help 54

6 Characteristics of CVI   61
　Two Sets of Traits   61
　Presentation of the Eyes   61
　Behavioral Presentations   63
7 The Thathachari's Journey with CVI   75
　In the Beginning   76
　Making Progress   78
　Relocating to Texas   79
　How to Cope   80
　Educational Methods   82
　My Inspirations   83
8 A Reason for Hope: Neuroplasticity   85
　Growing Evidence   85
　Enriched Environments and Synapse Strengthening   87
　Brain Trauma and Neuroplasticity—Intervention Can Help!   89
9 What to Do: Strategies for Helping Your Child Learn to See   93
　Strategies Must Be Functional   93
　Intervention Strategies   95
　Orientation Strategies   99
10 The Williams' Advocating   103
　Leah Williams' Story   103
　Leah's Educational Program—Managing the Shuffle   109
11 Moving Through Education Systems   113
　The Parent Is the First Teacher   113
　Team Members You May Meet along the Way   114
　Agreements among Team Members   115
　Individuals with Disabilities Education Act (IDEA)   117
　Transitioning from Early Intervention to Special Education   121
　After Age 5   122
Conclusion   125
About The Authors   127
Acknowledgements   129
Resources   131
Parent Support Groups   131
Blogs and Websites   131
Newsletters and Journals   132
Continuing Education and Information   133
Special Education Rights, Policies, and Assistance   134
ENDNOTES   139

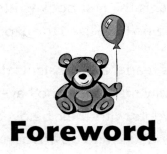

Foreword

By

Christine Roman-Lantzy, Ph.D.

In the 1970s and 1980s my first professional job was as a teacher of the visually impaired. I worked in the public school system as an itinerant teacher who traveled from school to school teaching visually impaired and blind children who were birth through 21 years of age. Some children attended their home school; others were in special education settings. One of my "schools" was actually a residential center for children who had multiple disabilities. It was in this center that I first encountered children who acted blind even though their medical histories had reports of normal eye exams. I attempted but failed to understand or intervene properly, but thoughts of these children and their mysterious form of visual impairment never left me.

Thankfully, parents, physicians, and educators now know more about CVI. We are still at the threshold of understanding the grand workings of vision in the brain, but in recent years there have been more research articles and books written to help doctors and teachers be more effective in diagnosing and educating children with CVI. And now thanks to Aubri Tallent, Andrei Tallent and Fredy Bush, there is also a resource written specifically to support families of children who have CVI. *Little Bear Sees* is the first book written about CVI from the perspective of parents who have lived the experience.

Little Bear Sees provides readers with insights that can only be offered by the parents and family members who have literally been through life and near-death events with their beloved children. They have ridden the rollercoaster of ups and downs as medical specialists have attached diagnoses to their children that might make even the most optimistic of us wonder if our children would ever experience the life we once dreamed for them. They have learned to navigate the extremely complex network of medical terminology, medication, seizure control and countless appointments. Parents have to learn an additional lexicon of terms associated with the educational system. Parents of children with CVI cannot simply send their child off to school; they have to digest the meanings of individualized educational programs, least restrictive environments, outcomes, goals, accommodations and specially designed instruction. They advocate for appropriate assessments, appropriate educational programs, appropriate equipment, and appropriate teachers. In short, parents have to become medical and educational experts.

Little Bear Sees is a book that provides both information and inspiration. It walks the reader through real family journeys and real family solutions. Parents who read *Little Bear Sees* will find a partner in their own experiences with the medical and educational challenges. The family stories may seem familiar and comforting. Parent-readers will appreciate the informational content that may fill in some of the gaps in their understanding of CVI. But this book should be read not only by families who experience CVI, it is equally important that the educational, medical, and therapy team members read *Little Bear Sees*. The most effective professionals are those who approach children with CVI with passion for the child and with a drive to learn about the subject. Aubri Tallent, Andrei Tallent, and Fredy Bush clearly under-stand this principle because *Little Bear Sees* is a book that informs the reader while also touching the heart.

CVI is now the leading cause of visual impairment in children who come from "first world" countries. It seems as though this large popu-lation of children appeared before physicians and educators were fully prepared to support their very special needs. This may be an explana-tion but it cannot be an excuse. Parents of children with CVI love their children no differently than those of us whose children do not have disabilities. Therefore, we are obligated to provide the children with CVI what any of us would want for our children—an opportunity to have the richest and best life possible. *Little Bear Sees* is a book that reminds all of us of the primacy of parents and the power of knowl-edge.

Christine Roman-Lantzy, Ph. D.
Author, *Cortical Visual Impairment: An Approach to Assessment and Intervention* (2007, AFB Press)

1
Little Bear Sees

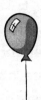

And you, a windrose, a compass, my direction,
my description of the world.

Ian Burgham

Meet Little Bear

Lukas Timothy Tallent (Little Bear) was born May 21, 2010. After eighteen hours of labor, Lukas came silently into this world. He did not take a breath and he did not cry. He was in his mother's arms for only seconds before he was whisked away, put on oxygen and transferred to the Neonatal Intensive Care Unit, or NICU. There he was put on a ventilator and hooked up to all kinds of wires, tubes and machines. It was hours before we got a chance to see him again, days before we were able to hold him and weeks before he finally came home.

While Lukas was in the NICU, we (his mom, dad and grandma) spent many hours watching him, talking to him, singing to him and holding him when we could. His mom, Aubri, sang her favorite childhood song, "Kookaburra," which was about an Australian bird whose call sounds like laughter. A line in the song is "Laugh Kookaburra, laugh Kookaburra, gay your life must be." Wanting to think of the laughter and happiness in Lukas' future, she began singing, "Laugh Lukas bear, laugh Lukas bear, gay your life will be." Eventually, Lukas' dad, Andrei, nicknamed him "Little Bear."

During the first week in the NICU, Lukas was diagnosed with Hypoxic Ischemic Encephalopathy (HIE), which meant that, essentially, at some point before birth he did not get enough oxygen. To this day, after countless doctors and specialists, no one can tell us exactly when, how or why this happened. We were told that he had also experienced bleeding in his brain and very likely had injury to his brain. He was quickly put on a cooling cap to help prevent further damage, which meant we watched our perfect little boy lie there for three days, necessarily sedated, and held his cold little hands as that was the only thing we could do.

An MRI several days later confirmed brain injury to many different areas of his brain. The doctors told us that they couldn't predict his future. It could be much better than it appeared or it could be much, much worse. We knew Lukas would likely be diagnosed with Cerebral Palsy in the future, but beyond that we didn't know what to expect. At times, we weren't sure if he would ever be able to come off the ventilator, breathe on his own, eat on his own, do anything much more than just lie there. After the six most difficult weeks of our lives, Lukas had opened his eyes, was breathing on his own, his seizures and high blood pressure were under control and we were able to bring him home. Lukas came home on a feeding tube, a million different medications, weekly nursing care, and with some scary unknowns about his future. We never lost sight, though, of how strong and brave our little boy was and we believed in him.

At the Beginning

At six weeks old, Lukas was young enough that we did not know yet how delayed in development he might be, but we did know one thing for sure: he did not look at us. In fact, he never seemed to look at much of anything. His eyes constantly darted around and did not seem to settle anywhere for more than a few seconds. In those early days, we were so overwhelmed trying to take care of our beautiful boy that worrying about his vision was certainly not a priority. We did not think there was much we could do and that it would just resolve on its own . . . or not.

At four months of age, our pediatrician suggested we take Lukas to an ophthalmologist. The ophthalmologist told us that Lukas could definitely see light, but there was no way to know what else he could see. He suggested that Lukas' vision may improve on its own, or it may not, but there was nothing we could do and no special toys we could buy to help him.

Wow, was he wrong! Today there is no question that our Little Bear can see. Lukas can see, and his vision improves every day. Today Lukas is a smiley, happy amazing little boy who looks at our faces, reaches for toys, is learning to operate a switch, can eat and drink orally and gets physically stronger all the time.

At seven months of age, an amazing teacher for the visually impaired (TVI), Kymberlee Gilkey, came to see Lukas through our Early Intervention program. She told us that Lukas showed signs of cortical visual impairment (CVI). Upon hearing this, we felt a range of emotions. We were afraid at what that might mean for his future. We were confused about why no one had mentioned this before, and we were relieved to finally have a place to start searching for information. We want to share with you what we have learned about CVI and what you can do to help your child learn to see.

Fitting Puzzle Pieces Together for Little Bear

After Kymberlee left, we immediately searched the internet for more information. We found bits and pieces scattered across a variety of websites, but nothing that really told us what we urgently needed to know: will it get better, and what do we do? We did order and read *Cortical Visual Impairment: An Approach to Assessment and Intervention* by Christine Roman-Lantzy. We had no idea then how this book and Dr. Roman-Lantzy would change our lives. When the book arrived, we scanned its pages for answers to those urgent questions. Much of the information was there, but it seemed buried among a lot of technical language that we were not ready to process. We needed a quick-start guide; we desperately wanted to know where to start and what to expect. We wanted to know about other families, what they were doing and how it was helping their children. We wanted to hear stories of success!

Before we knew that Lukas had CVI, we were told by various people to use black and white with him. We were encouraged to show him pictures and surround him with toys that were primarily black and white. Once we started to learn about CVI, we discovered that black and white is entirely inappropriate for kids with CVI. Typically, they can see bright, saturated colors like fire engine red or sunshine yellow much more easily than black and white. We also learned that kids with CVI often have a preferred color, usually red or yellow, which can be used in the beginning to stimulate their vision. We tried different colors and found that Lukas also really responded to red and yellow. The first time we showed him his red Elmo doll, he looked at it, opened his mouth and laughed. We had never before seen him react so clearly to something he saw. Elmo and Big Bird became fixtures in our daily routine.

Using what we learned from our TVI, a few key websites, and Dr.

Roman-Lantzy's book, we began to piece together a plan to help Lukas' vision improve. As with so many aspects of caring for Lukas, it was a steep learning curve in the beginning. We had to learn how to interpret his visual behaviors and how to adapt the environment to give him every opportunity to see. He didn't look at things the way we expected him to. When something caught his attention, it often took him some time before he would look. When he did look, he would glance at it very briefly before looking away. We learned to be patient. We learned that, if he continued to glance back at it, this meant he was seeing it. Every time his gaze returned to an object, he was strengthening those connections in his brain and improving his vision.

We learned that we needed to keep things simple by adding black backgrounds and reducing any visual or other sensory clutter, like background noises that might distract him. We made sure not to make any noise when presenting him with an object to look at. We made sure, in the beginning, that the objects were only one color and that there was always a black background behind them.

We learned that movement was a great way to get Lukas' attention. We found various ways to incorporate movement into his visual world. When showing him Elmo, we would make him dance. We found that shiny materials mimic movement and so we bought bright red or yellow Mylar balloons that would sparkle in the sunlight. We would place the string in his hand so that he could watch the balloons move as he moved.

We learned that using light was another way to help Lukas see. We found brightly colored glow sticks that he could hold in his hands. Our vision teacher brought a light box to help illuminate objects he was looking at. We began to research iPad apps that he could see, since the iPad is backlit. Eventually, we even created an app specifically for kids with CVI that Lukas loves.

We tried placing objects in different parts of his field of vision and at different distances from him to understand how he could see best. We found that it was difficult for him to see anything below his face and easier if objects were placed on the left side. We found that closer was always easier, but that he could see certain things up to about three feet.

Creating a Vision Routine

When Lukas was eleven months old, we heard that Dr. Roman-Lantzy was coming to Honolulu to give a talk! We were incredibly excited and signed up right away. A few weeks before her arrival, we were told that she would be able to see a handful of kids during her trip and were asked if we wanted her to see Lukas. What a blessing this was! We were thrilled at the opportunity!

We learned so much during her talk, but it was really that one-on-one session that gave us considerable insight and more hope for Lukas. She verified that Lukas did indeed display characteristics of CVI, and she assessed him to be in the very early stages of Phase II. (You can learn more about Dr. Roman's method of assessment and the phases of CVI in chapter 6.)

From Dr. Roman-Lantzy, we learned that the best thing we could do to help Lukas learn to see was not to think of vision activities as therapy. We had to find ways to incorporate opportunities for him to see into his everyday life. She had stressed that frequency was far more important than duration. We couldn't just set aside an hour a day to work on vision, but instead had to adapt Lukas' world so that he could use his vision all day long.

She told us about a study she had done which found that in a select group of children with CVI, who had highly motivated parents, 97% went from Phase I to Phase III, or near normal vision, in an average of 3.7 years. She gave us some great ideas on how to continue helping him, and she told us that she saw so much potential in him! We were inspired!

After meeting with her, we immediately began to implement some of her suggestions. We hung shiny red objects by Lukas' changing table and car seat so that he would begin to have a visual association with those parts of his daily routine. We added bright red slap bracelets and ribbon to his bottles. We created a sparkly red heart out of craft foam and pipe cleaner to attach to his spoon during meals. We added bright red butterflies to his stroller so that he could watch them bounce along everywhere we went. We took Elmo with us everywhere because we had learned that familiar objects are easier for kids with CVI to identify and look at than novel objects.

Once Little Bear got good at seeing red and yellow, we began to introduce new colors. We bought those same shiny Mylar balloons in blue and purple. We began placing shiny pink beads against that black background instead of red or yellow and immediately we saw him reach for them. We discovered that Lukas likes pink even better than red! We found a bright pink lei that we hung next to him during his physical therapy. We bought a bright pink stuffed monkey that became a constant companion. We learned that we have to be persistent, to just keep trying because we never know when something will click and we'll see another side of Lukas we didn't know was there.

Our daily routine begins with changing his diaper and clothes. As we do this, Lukas likes to look at and reach for the shiny red snowflake hanging on the wall. After that, we feed him his breakfast out of a bright red bowl using a spoon with a shiny red heart attached, so he can always see it coming towards him. He drinks from a bottle with a shiny red slap bracelet wrapped around it. Before we begin feeding him, we make sure to show him the bottle or spoon while we say, "Are you ready to eat? Here's your spoon, here's your bottle."

After breakfast, Lukas heads to Grandma's house, which is just down the street and is much larger than our apartment, to begin his therapies. He does physical therapy for three hours, five days a week. He also often has appointments with various Early Intervention therapists, such as occupational, speech, vision, or nutrition. In between his various therapies, we take breaks for naps or to have lunch. We use the same visual routine for lunch and dinner as we do for breakfast. While Lukas is digesting, we often show him one of his favorite objects and have him practice looking, holding, reaching for and touching it.

In the evenings, we usually spend some time with the light box or iPad, which are great visual activities after dark. We may put him in his high chair and have him practice turning the light box on and off with his switch or hold him and show him some of his favorite iPad apps so that he can practice reaching. These are great visual tasks that also incorporate cause and effect and motor skills. He also really enjoys them!

Before bed, we usually give Lukas some time to just lay on the sofa or bed and play. This is the position he likes best. If we have balloons in the house, we will place these nearby so that he can look at them and hold them or bat at them. Another favorite toy is a red cascade centerpiece from the party store. We tuck the base of it under his torso so he can watch it shake every time he moves his arms or legs. Other times we will skip the visual activities and just talk or sing to him. He loves to vocalize along with our singing and reach out to touch our faces. These are some of the most precious moments in our day.

Today, Lukas is almost two years old and has made an unbelievable amount of progress! We know he is learning and growing and changing all time. We can't imagine where he would be now if it weren't for everything we have learned along the way about how to help his vision. In 2011, we created our company, Little Bear Sees, with the idea of doing everything we could to help spread the word about CVI. We started with a website, www.LittleBearSees.org, then an iPad app, Tap-n-See Zoo™, and now this book. We know that many families are still being told there is nothing they can do to help their children learn to see. We want you to know that our children can learn to see!

Why We Wrote this Book

Securing knowledge, accurate information, and personal and professional support can seem nearly impossible when your child has cortical visual impairment. Many doctors seem to know very little about CVI, and resources that do exist are not written for parents. We wanted to know exactly what CVI was and what we could do about it. We eventually found the information that we are presenting to you in this book, and that gave us hope. Hope is the most important thing we want to pass on to you.

We are the authors, Aubri, Andrei and Fredy, mother, father and grandmother respectively of Lukas. As a result of our many experiences and challenges in finding solutions, we have become a family team and advocates for Lukas. Together, we educated ourselves, sought help and developed a program to train Lukas' brain to translate what he sees. We created this book to give you all the resources, information and hope that we wish had been easy to find in our search. In this book, we want to help you understand CVI and how to organize an action plan for your child that will make a significant difference in her vision.

As Lukas' grandmother, I had several emotional responses upon hearing the diagnosis. My heart sank. I wondered about his future. I had so many questions: How is he going to learn? To interact? How is he going to communicate? His eyes are so important, even basic to seeing my face, his parents' smiles and rolling across a room. After we learned more about CVI, I became angry because I realized that we could have left Lukas very visually impaired if we had given up. With my family, I turned my emotional energy into action.

When Lukas was four months old, we were told that there was no way to know how much he could see and that there was nothing we could do to help him. We knew that Lukas could see more than just light and we believed he had a lot of potential. Many of the people we have met have children who were either not diagnosed, or misdiagnosed, and often were told that their child could not see, and there was nothing they could do. The statement that we could do nothing was appalling, frightening, and made us angry enough to say, "We don't believe it."

"I Don't Believe It" Responses Are Good

Parents tend to think that the doctors are right and so will not question, research, or even go against a diagnosis. They are the professionals after all. The neurologist did not tell us that Lukas had CVI. The ophthalmologist told us to wait and see. There were so many opportunities early on for people to say, "He possibly has CVI, and there is a lot you can do." If it had not been for the teacher of the visually impaired (TVI) we met when Lukas was seven months old, who knows how long it would have taken for us to learn about CVI? To this day, no doctor has ever officially diagnosed Lukas with CVI.

Yet, this thought remained on our minds and spurred us to share what we know: Imagine how we would feel if Lukas were five years old, and we were just learning about CVI.

Our hope with this book is to get the information out to as many parents as possible with this **critical message:** Our children can see AND they can learn to see. We can teach their brains how to interpret what their eyes can see. In fact, there is so much we can do.

Here is what motivates us...In our experience, we have met many families with children whose brains have not been taught to interpret what their eyes are seeing, and that virtually renders them functionally blind. We are hoping that you will help us prevent this from happening by giving this book to other parents who need it. In addition to this book, you can find further information about CVI and tips for helping your child on www.LittleBearSees.org. We have also established "Little Bear Sees," a non-profit organization geared towards providing families in need with the information, products, and tools to help their children with CVI learn to see.

We believe that vision is a primary foundational piece of our lives, and yet, kids with CVI are not getting the help they need because they are not getting diagnosed. If they are diagnosed and intervention takes place, their vision will improve. The fact that many children are either misdiagnosed or not diagnosed at all is tragic and avoidable.

What You Will Learn

In the following pages, we will discuss what CVI is, the primary characteristics of CVI, the research around neuroplasticity, and offer information and strategies to help your child learn to see. In addition to our family, we will introduce three other families whose stories will demonstrate the progress children can make with family focus and vision intervention. You can make such a difference!

Contrary to many doctors' opinions, the brain will continue to change and can be taught, even into adulthood. Professionals working with kids who have CVI understand that teaching the brain to see and building the neural pathways should start as early as possible, when the brain is most pliable in visual development. The education of the brain continues with appropriate techniques for developing visual skills that are integrated into daily routines like bath time, eating and playing. With this intervention, many of these children will improve their ability to distinguish or make sense of what they see. Early intervention is best, but it is NEVER too late to begin!

Now you understand that we wrote *Little Bear Sees* to make sure that children are not being left functionally blind from a lack of education. Our desire is to educate you, comfort you, and give you hope.

We also hope that you will spread the word to teachers of the visually impaired, ophthalmologists, educators, healthcare workers, early intervention workers and other parents. The more people who understand our children and interact with them appropriately, the better!

2

The Importance of Family and Bonding

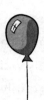

You've developed the strength of a draft horse while holding onto the delicacy of a daffodil . . . you are the mother, advocate and protector of a child with a disability.

Lori Borgman

The Importance of Family

The commitment on the part of the family to help a child learn to see is vital. As we discussed in chapter 1, incorporating many opportunities for your child to use vision in her daily routine is crucial. To do this successfully, all caregivers in a child's life should be committed to that goal. Yes, it takes time, but, as you will see in chapter 9, the therapy and activities are not difficult. Our role as Lukas' family has been to teach his brain to start interpreting the data his eyes see. We are constantly stimulating Lukas' brain to do its work.

In order to help Lukas, we had to learn as much as possible about CVI and we had to learn Lukas' behaviors and ways of communicating what he could see. We had to learn, and teach others in his world, to give him time to look at an object, to simplify what we wanted him to look at and to give him lots of opportunities to see whether he was engaged in eating, getting his diaper changed, doing physical therapy or just playing. We discovered that, like many children with CVI, Lukas initially responded best to red. We filled his world with bright red objects so that he could easily use his vision throughout the day.

Once we began to realize how much of a difference we could make in Lukas' vision, we were stunned that any doctor would tell us to simply "wait and see." If we merely waited to see if Lukas' vision would improve on its own, it most certainly would not have improved. By listening to the doctors, we could have created severe visual impairment in our child.

We want you to know how important vision is in motivating children to want to learn, to grasp, to connect, and to move. Visual function will improve and resolve if there is consistent daily intervention. Little Lukas, who rarely looked at us for the first year of his life, is now looking at our faces, balloons, toys, books and many other things. His world is opening up.

The Importance of Bonding

There are few words we can say to express the depth of joy and inspiration we have found in bonding with and learning with Lukas. That is not to say that, like any new parents and grandparents, we have not been sleep deprived, felt exhausted and numb, and wondered how we could best assist our beautiful son. Yes, we worried, dreamed, cried, and searched for answers. What we did as new parents was to remember that this baby also needed bonding, empathy and touch to welcome him to his new life, help him integrate his sensory awareness, and learn how to adapt to his new environment.

Our natural inclination was to connect however we could. It has been difficult to not be able to connect with him through eye contact. However, by touching Lukas in a comforting way, holding him, rocking him, talking to him and singing to him, we knew we were stimulating the growth of his brain to integrate nerve impulses. Touch, movement and sound, accompanied by a loving, emotional connection, helped each of us with our stress levels.

Eventually, we learned to follow our instincts about how to support Lukas. In fact, according to Dr. Roman-Lantzy, your instincts as a parent play an integral role in reading your child's cues and knowing their needs, especially when you cannot look into their eyes for those connecting moments. She refers to the work of Selma Fraiberg, a psychoanalyst, author, and pioneer in the field of infant psychiatry, as another way to bond with your child without eye contact. According to Dr. Roman-Lantzy, Selma Fraiberg "was a psychologist at the University of Michigan who studied bonding between parent and child, when the child was born blind or significantly vision impaired. The problem was that the kids did not make eye contact with their parents, but she learned that children would move their hands, especially in ways that communicated how they are feeling. So a clenched fist or splayed open fingers would be different expressions. She taught parents that their child was giving them cues."

Dr. Roman-Lantzy emphasizes that, "It is really important for families to know that if your child does not look at you, it does not mean that they are not bonded to you. It does not mean that they are rejecting you. It does not mean they do not love and need you and you them. It just feels a little bit different. I think parents find it as an extremely big obstacle that kids with CVI do not look into their parents' faces for many years and sometimes never at all. That is because the part of their brain that regulates facial recognition and all that complexity is injured."

"It is so important that family members understand their child while they are holding them and cuddling with them and having those bonding experiences with them. In those moments, they can watch how their baby moves, and how their baby moves toward them, and watch how the baby feels more relaxed in their arms than anybody else's arms. They have to trust their instincts in interpreting their child's actions and movements."[1]

Dr. Roman-Lantzy shares, "Parents can allow themselves to believe their child can do and grow and be more. When they are observing their child, it is also important that they understand that what they instinctually feel, what they think, what they are seeing . . . they should trust those instincts."[2]

Many parents are told that either their child's vision is fine, though they know it is not, or that their vision is impaired, but there is nothing they can do. Parents are often the first to believe that this is not true. They know their child's vision is not typical, but they believe they can make a difference.

Those observations often fall flat on the ears of doctors, but as Dr. Roman-Lantzy observes, "Parents can push through the objections and say, 'I'm going to find somebody who will believe me.' That's really important. They have to believe in themselves and in their observations."[3]

Follow the Child's Lead

Lukas' Grandmother, Fredy, shared that the family's program for Lukas grew based upon their observations of Lukas and deciphering the clues he gave them. Fredy shares: "It doesn't take long before you recognize what your child prefers to look at, how they look, and what they more readily look at versus what's harder for them to look at. Our understanding of Lukas started with our intuition to watch, observe, and adapt. Each parent has to discover how her child with CVI learns to see. Because Lukas had a lot of brain injury, that typical process was gone. We had to figure out how we could get his brain to start communicating and encourage his brain to start interpreting."

"For example, Lukas took to red right away, and then the next toy he took to was yellow, and from there it was blue rather than the orange color that I thought it might be. But your child shows you. It's so important to pay attention to this. Helping a child with CVI is not about trying to make them see things that are more complex. It's about learning what they can see and then providing opportunities for them to look at something with each part of their day, so there's always an opportunity to learn to see. Eventually, their ability to see more complexity will come."

"In observing Lukas, we realized that he was completely uninterested in objects with too many colors or patterns, and we could never get him interested in them. Our goal wasn't to find a way to make him interested, but instead to see what did interest his brain. What made him look and be curious? After focusing for so long on red and yellow, we recently gave him this bright, shiny, plastic pink lei. It's very bright pink, and to our surprise, he loves it. He talks to it. He laughs with it. We had no idea that he would like pink. One of us happened to pick it up, and as soon as he saw it, he responded to it. So the journey is very intuitive and we are always watching to see how our child responds."

Fredy continues, "When we saw how excited he was about pink, we bought more toys that were bright pink and we started introducing more pink into his daily routine because he loves it so much. We followed Lukas' lead in this regard. If we did not do this, his vision would not be improving like it is."

"Think of all of the areas that are affected by eyesight. So in other words, children with CVI don't reach for toys because they don't see. If they don't reach for toys, they don't learn textures. If they don't reach for toys, they don't learn their fine motor skills. If they can't see your face, they're not curious outside their own body. They don't see that they're in a much bigger space or room, so they don't have a need to crawl, especially if they're well taken care of. They're happy, and they're being fed, and they're getting their naps, and they're being loved. They don't have a desire to walk, because they don't see the other side of the room. The ability to see impacts both physical and cognitive development. If we didn't follow Lukas' lead, he wouldn't be able to overcome these challenges. He wouldn't learn to see."

The Defining Moments

Lukas' dad, Andrei, had a defining moment in finally connecting to Lukas. "Once I was able to hold Lukas without him being hooked up to an IV, a ventilator and a feeding tube, that was my defining moment when I did not feel like we were disconnected, when I could be one with him. That was a big thing for me. Lukas does not make eye contact because of CVI, and that was really difficult for me because I think eye contact is a very intimate thing. I think the lack of that made it difficult to bond early on. So being able to hold him was a wonderful feeling . . . to be able to connect with him in that way, rather than with eye contact, was my gift."

Keeping the Faith

Lukas' mom, Aubri, found comfort in other ways. "Whenever it all became too much, I would ask myself what I was grateful for in that moment. I could always find something, such as Lukas' smile, the feeling of his weight in my arms, the fact that he is here with us. These things helped keep me in the present and let go of all my future concerns. Partly you just keep going because you have to. Lukas is my absolute inspiration. If he can go through everything he has had to go through in his life so far and still smile every day, then so can I.

Connecting with other parents and hearing their stories and ideas, particularly parents who are further down the road than we are, also helps to give me that hope and faith. In one parenting group, they refer to the progress their children make as inchstones rather than milestones. This is a great way to focus on what I am thankful for. Lukas is doing new things all the time that we were never certain he'd be able to do. He may not be meeting all those milestones, but he is meeting hundreds of inchstones and, eventually, I am confident he will get there."

Lukas' Grandmother's Inspiration

Fredy shares her journey with Lukas thus far: "I don't think anyone's ever touched me as deeply as Lukas does, ever. He's courageous, and he's dealing with things that I'll never have to deal with. He's always smiling. He works hard every day, whether it's the physical therapy or the occupational therapy. There is a spark in Lukas that wants to move, to know, and to see, and I think that must be inherent to the human spirit. Loving Lukas, who bravely faces so many challenges every day, touches my heart deeply. I mean he laughs and he smiles, and he just doesn't know that it should be any different, that most kids don't work out three hours a day, and have a hard time seeing. He is one of the greatest gifts in my life. I don't think I've ever done anything in my life that's meant more to me than spending the last two years with him. He doesn't give up and neither will we. We have never accepted the word 'no.' We believe that he can and will achieve so much more. There is no rule. There is only the love we share, the way we decipher his clues and his seeing, and knowing intuitively what our next step is to support Lukas."

Other moms of children with CVI have found their strength in other ways and will share their words of inspiration with you in the following pages.

Krista's Advocacy

The Williams family, Krista and Brandon, and their children Noah, Elijah and Leah have faced similar challenges. You can read more about their story in chapter 10.

Six years ago, when Leah was born, Krista Williams worked Monday through Friday and Brandon Williams was working three twelve-hour shifts Saturdays through Mondays. Since Brandon was home during the week, he was Leah's primary caregiver. Six months after Leah's diagnosis of CVI and infantile spasms, Krista chose to quit her job and to stay home with Leah. Noah was the only one in school at the time. They were doing his homework either late at night or early in the morning before he went to school. Krista knew the boys were getting pushed aside, and it was not a good thing. Noah was in school, little Elijah was just turning three, and little Leah was now receiving in-home vision therapy, physical therapy and occupational therapy. The family had a full schedule.

We asked Krista how she stayed inspired and focused.

Krista shares, "How do I stay inspired? Well, Leah was never supposed to even be able to sit up by herself, and she walks all over the place. Thank God we had awesome doctors who never gave us a bleak outlook. After the fact, they said, 'She shouldn't be doing this.'"

"My inspiration is to get Leah as far as she can go. Let her achieve as much as she possibly can. She is never going to be a typical girl, and I want her to be able to do as much as she can for herself, and I will be with her every step of the way to make sure that happens. She has inspired us more by her pushing through. She is very stubborn, but I think that that is an advantage for her. When she would crawl underneath our rocking chair and could not get out, I did not pull her out. I let her try because if we are there all the time doing things for her, she is never going to learn to do things on her own. The hardest thing is knowing where Leah's actual limitations are and how far we should push her. You have to observe. Everything is observation."

"I would not let her go to the point of frustration where there was no getting her back, but finding that line is still observation. She has surprised me at the things she can do. I am telling you, one of the best things was getting the girl an iPad. I would have thought she was lower functioning than what she really is because I did not know what was inside that her learning on the iPad brings out. The iPad motivates her. She likes it. She likes the reward. She likes the sound. Her visual attention has increased."

"Do not give up and keep pushing your child. They can do a lot more. You have to advocate. If you do not advocate, they may get nowhere. If you do not push the child and keep educating her, you will never know what she can do. Aim high! These kids are capable of a lot more than what we all realize."

Kevin and Alicia's Emotional Roller Coaster

Kevin and Alicia Champine of Marysville, Washington are parents of 16-month-old Carson, who you will read more about in chapter 5. In the beginning, Alicia and Kevin were unsure of how long Carson was going to live. The prognosis made it hard for Kevin to fully bond. He held Carson, loved him and cared for him, but his guard was up because he was so afraid to get more emotionally attached than he already was. After all, Carson was his only son. Alicia learned over time that a lot of fathers struggle with this in the beginning.

The motherly instinct for Alicia's bonding started immediately with breastfeeding Carson. Yet, within several months, that true bond between father and son developed. Alicia notes that while she wanted to push Kevin's bonding, she did not want him to put a wall up when she suggested that he not worry about what is down the road.

Kevin and Alicia understand that each of them had to deal with their own emotions. From the very beginning, they allowed each other to feel as they did without judgment or questioning or making each other feel bad. They struggled together during the pregnancy, and neither wanted to drive a wedge in their relationship.

Alicia says, "We allow and accept. There were times when one person would say what was on their mind, and the other did not quite get it or feel the same way. We might not have understood, but we simply acknowledged, 'Okay, that is how you are feeling. I accept that.'"

"When you first learn about a child's disabilities or medical conditions, emotions are running so high and so intense. It seems like the safest person to be able to share those feelings with would be the other parent because they are in the midst of it with you. If you are making the other person feel bad about their emotions, thoughts or feelings, you are going to end up not talking to each other. You are going to feel like you are going through it alone."

"Kevin did not have a lot of people with whom to talk. Both my parents are still around, and they are emotionally supportive people for me. I met with the nurse and I got the chance to talk with her and the therapist. I was Kevin's go-to person, and I was like an open place for him to be able to speak his emotions because men have such a tendency to shut down emotionally and not want to talk about it. I needed to be as open as possible so that he could speak the things that he was feeling. It is like if nobody else is there, we have to be there for each other."

"We do not have any other friends who have kids with any sort of medical conditions. I need to be able to be his sounding board and a person to talk to. That would definitely be an encouragement that I would give to parents beginning their CVI journey—to allow each other to be able to speak and mull over what has happened."

"We are now sixteen months into this journey. Even now, most of the time, our days are normal and natural for us. Therapy with Carson is now a part of our day, like anybody else who may go for a walk every day. Then there are days where, for whatever reason, you have one hard day and need to share. For example, I say each month that Carson's eight months old or Carson's twelve months old. Well on this last monthly birthday at sixteen months, for some reason that number was difficult for me. To me, sixteen months of age was the difference between Carson being a baby and being a toddler. On Sunday, I was down. I felt like all day I was on the verge of tears. And I did not have a lot of energy throughout the day."

"Most days are just 'normal' life with joy and smiles, schedules, discipline, diapers to change, meals to make. Then we hit these one-day grieving periods out of the blue. A few months ago, one of our friends had a baby boy. We knew it was a boy and we were so excited. The day the baby was born, we went through a time of grieving, grieving for what we had envisioned for our son and us. I think that may be the best advice for parents who are up and coming. Any parent of a child with any sort of special needs should understand that grief can creep on, the smallest event or thought can trigger it, and they can have a plan for those hard days. The other special needs parents I have ever talked to know it is such a normal reaction. It is not bad that you go through these normal emotions and feelings of grief, sadness, or discouragement."

"I grieve because I want the absolute best for Carson. I grieve because things did not work out the way that I had thought or envisioned. None of us as mothers want to see our kids struggle, ever. We want them to be happy and whole and everything to work out perfectly for them because having a child with special needs means they struggle more. So it is okay to grieve and I do not feel guilty about those grieving times because I know that I love him. I bond with him and I give of myself to him."

"The truth is, regardless of those struggles, Carson is the happiest child I have ever been around. He is a happy, easy-going, loving child. I think sometimes we do focus so much on the therapies, the doctor's appointments, the struggles, that we have to stop and to soak that in for a little bit and let ourselves go. They are happy and enjoy that moment. I think that is important."

The Champine's honesty in dealing with such overwhelming circumstances is real and true for most families who care or will care for a child with special needs. All of us pass through stages of grief and deal with emotional overload. It is important to know that these feelings are common and you are not alone.

Signs of the Blues and Depression

In dealing with grief and all that it takes to parent a special needs child, you may find yourself struggling with depression. New mothers are often at risk for post-partum depression by virtue of the stress and hormone fluctuations of having a new baby. Parents of children with disabilities are known to be at greater risk for depression.[4] Parental depression can interfere with the development of attachment that is critical for a child's social and emotional development.[5] If this is something you are struggling with, know that you are not alone. We will discuss it briefly below to help you find the support and care that you need.

Most moms experience mood swings and the "blues" after having a baby. This moodiness is normal and is caused by the surges of hormones, exhaustion and process of adjusting to having a new baby.

General symptoms for the blues, which is not depression, include:

- Mood swings
- General tension or anxiety
- Sadness
- Irritability
- Crying
- Trouble sleeping

Even general depression can be normal, particularly when you're faced with the many challenges of caring for a child with special needs and is in no way a character flaw or defect. The reason we suggest you watch for the deeper signs of depression is that once the biochemistry of depression becomes anchored in your body and brain, the situation becomes more difficult to deal with. Depression symptoms include:

- Loss of appetite
- Insomnia
- Intense irritability and anger
- Overwhelming fatigue
- Loss of interest in sex
- Lack of joy in life
- Feelings of shame, guilt or inadequacy
- Severe mood swings
- Thoughts of harming yourself or your child
- Difficulty bonding with your child
- Withdrawal from family and friends[6]

You cannot deal with depression alone. You need support because it is very easy to make the slide downhill from general anxiety to all-out depression. Left untreated, depression can interfere with your ability to bond and care for your child. Finding someone to talk to, such as a parenting group, a parenting coach or counselor, or a mental health expert such as a therapist or psychiatrist, can be a good first step. A medical doctor or psychiatrist can also help you by prescribing an anti-depressant medication. We hope you take this section to heart and allow yourself the same care and love you give to your child. Reach out and seek support. Ask for help. You may be surprised at the love and support that comes back to you.

3

Cortical Visual Impairment

Traditionally, educators for the visually impaired assisted only those whose eye conditions were associated with visual loss (reduced acuity). Now it has become necessary to offer services for those whose visual loss is due to brain damage. Thus, the definition of CVI was born.

Dr. James E Jan

What is Cortical Visual Impairment (CVI)?

Cortical visual impairment (CVI) is a neurological disorder in which there is damage to the posterior visual pathways and/or the occipital lobes of the brain resulting in visual processing issues. The inability to process visual information is a form of visual impairment, but what exactly is it? Can it be corrected with glasses or surgery? Under-standing what CVI is and what it is not helps us realize which interventions will be most effective.

In the past, vision problems were mostly defined as loss in acuity (how far the eyes can see) and/or severe visual field loss (a blind area in the peripheral vision). Researchers and doctors knew that there was more to visual impairment, but they used those definitions in order to help adults with visual impairment get the social assistance they needed. The definition was limiting by virtue of not including or addressing the visual impairments of children that occur for different reasons.[7]

Cortical visual impairment has often been referred to by other terms, including cerebral visual impairment, neurological visual impairment, cortical blindness, and brain injury-related visual impairment. All of these terms refer to visual dysfunction resulting from injury to visual centers of the brain. In this book, we will refer to it as cortical visual impairment or CVI. Dr. Roman-Lantzy, author of the book *Cortical Visual Impairment*, explains that the term cortical blindness was established for adults who had heart attacks and occasionally had this temporary form of blindness after a period of anoxia (absence of oxygen to an organ or tissue). "The term cortical visual impairment is *more* appropriate than the term cortical blindness because there really are no children in the CVI category who are totally blind."[8] Cortical blindness suggests a permanent inability to see, whereas children with CVI can learn to see over time!

As we will discuss further in chapter 4, vision is not just one process, but a combination of events. When a person looks at an object, light rays are taken into the eyes where they hit the rods and cones in the retina. The light causes chemical changes in those cells and is converted to electrical energy. The electrical signals travel through the optic nerve to the visual cortex area of the brain and convert the signals to images that have meaning. In other words, the job of the visual cortex of the brain is to make sense of the image it receives from the eyes. Without proper functioning in this area of the brain, typical vision cannot occur. Children with CVI may additionally have other visual impairments, but they also may have normal acuity and field of vision.

CVI is a specific type of visual impairment that relates to how the brain processes visual information, and this can develop and change over time depending upon intervention and the child's adaptability to her environment. Because of this, glasses or surgery will not correct CVI. Your child may still need glasses as a result of some other eye condition, but they will not correct CVI.

What Causes CVI?

CVI is caused by widespread injury to the areas of the brain that are responsible for the sense of vision. According to Dr. Roman-Lantzy, common conditions associated with or contributing to CVI include:

• Asphyxia - oxygen deprivation

• Perinatal hypoxic-ischemic encephalopathy—too little oxygen disrupts the blood flow causing reduced flow to the brain

• Traumatic head injury

• Structural abnormalities—any disruption in the normal growth process that has significant neurological consequences

• Cerebral vascular accident or stroke

• Periventricular Leukomalacia (PVL) damage and softening of the white matter

• Intraventricular hemorrhage, bleeding into the brain's ventricular system, the brain's structures which hold the cerebral spinal fluid

• Infections inside the uterus during gestation or infections that are acquired after birth

While it is important to understand what causes CVI, it is even more vital to identify it as early as possible so that treatment and education can begin.

How Many Children Have CVI?

In response to the question of the incidence of CVI, researchers agree that the number of people with CVI is growing. Dr. Roman-Lantzy states that, "CVI is the leading cause of visual impairment in children from first-world countries today. As medicine advances, more people, particularly children, with neurological injury are surviving. As more survivors of brain injury live, many go on to develop CVI."[9]

Exact numbers of children with CVI are hard to come by, in part because it is so often undiagnosed or misdiagnosed. Researchers, however, can offer some insight through their statistics. "A variety of studies indicate the percentage of children with vision impairments who have CVI is between 3.6 and 21%, making it the major cause of vision impairment in children."[10] In a study from Liverpool, Rogers found that CVI was the most common cause of visual impairment in children with associated neurological disorders (49% of the study population). In Northern California, CVI was also found to be the leading cause of visual impairment in children under the age of five years.[11]

In summary, what global researchers can document in varied regions is that the number of children with a CVI diagnosis is increasing, and they anticipate this trend to continue. Additionally, CVI is rarely the only diagnosis a child has. A study conducted by Maryke Groenveld, Ph.D. R.Psych., found that a large percentage of children with CVI had, "cerebral palsy (about 80%), epilepsy (about 60%), hydrocephalus (about 20%) and deafness (about 10%)."[12]

Diagnosis

With so many children affected by CVI, you might wonder how the condition is diagnosed. The diagnosis of CVI can be made in the doctor's office, but often it is not. Extensive brain scans and other tests add information to the diagnosis, but the best situation is a doctor conducting a thorough examination of the child and gathering information about the child's history of any event or process that might have contributed to brain injury.

Unfortunately, many doctors still do not know much about CVI and may not know what to look for. We know of many families whose children were not diagnosed with CVI until they had learned about it and convinced their doctors that this is what their child had.

A child with CVI might have a normal eye exam. If your child has had a normal eye exam, and you still think something is wrong, keep observing your child, keep track of and write down behaviors found in checklists in chapter 6. When you talk to a doctor or other health professional, they may be distracted or pass off your concerns. Be persistent.

You live with your child, and you know your child. Take a notebook with your observations to any doctor's appointment, and ask the health professional to review your list. Then there is an opportunity for discussion. Your writing shows that you are a concerned parent, and that you are not going away. Be a champion for your child and educate your doctor, who may not always have answers. Because many doctors are not trained to look for CVI, it is often unnoticed.

It is important to realize, however, that even without an official diagnosis, you can still begin intervention. We first heard about CVI from Lukas' TVI, Kymberlee Gilkey. Dr. Roman-Lantzy later confirmed the presence of CVI characteristics in Lukas, but none of his doctors have ever given an official diagnosis. Despite this, we have learned about CVI, observed those presenting characteristics in Lukas and found ways to help him improve his vision. We'll introduce the common characteristics of CVI next.

Characteristics of CVI

Many children with CVI share some common characteristics. Knowing these can help you to spot if your child might have CVI. Your child may have all or just some of these characteristics. We will outline them below and discuss them more thoroughly in chapter 6.

Appearance

• Does not look blind

• Blank facial expression

• Lack of visual communication skills

• Eye movements smooth, but aimless

• Nystagmus (rapid eye movement or rhythmic, involuntary eye movement horizontally)

Visual Function

• Visual function appears to vary from day to day or hour to hour

• Has limited visual attention and lack of visual curiosity

• Is aware of distant objects, but not able to identify

• Spontaneous visual activity has short duration

• May require some time before visually engaging an object

• Tires easily from visual activities

• Closes eyes or turns away while listening

• Balance improves with eyes closed

• Looks away from people and objects

• Consistently looks to either side when using vision

• When visually reaching, looks with a slight downward gaze

• Turns head to side when reaching, as if using peripheral fields

• Prefers items of a specific color, such as red or yellow

• Prefers shiny objects or objects that move, such as a pinwheel

• Has difficulty with visual complexity

• Tends to gaze at lights or stare without purpose

• Visual blink reflex is absent or impaired

• Prefers familiar objects over new ones

• Uses touch to identify objects

Mobility Skills

• Occasionally sees better traveling in a car

• Has difficulties with depth perception, inaccurate reach

• Unable to estimate distances

• Has difficulties with spatial interpretation

• Avoids obstacles, but is unable to use vision for close work

Improved Visual Performance

• When in familiar environments and when using familiar objects

• When the environment is quiet and free of distractions

• When told "what" to look for and "where" to look

• When objects are held close to the eyes when viewing

• When objects are widely spaced

• When looking at one object versus a group of objects

• When color is used to assist in identification of objects or shapes

• When in a comfortable position that is not physically demanding

• When objects are against a plain background and paired with movement or light[13]

If your child has some or many of these symptoms, it is necessary to look at your child's history. Was it a normal pregnancy? Was there another problem with the child's brain at birth (such as hydro-cephalus, cysts, or other malformations)? Did the child have high fevers, meningitis, or a metabolic disorder? Was there a near-drowning incident, some other accident or a traumatic brain injury that may not have been diagnosed at the time?

Here are some of the tests that provide additional information to help in the diagnosis of CVI:

- An ERG (Electroretinogram) may be requested to rule out retinal problems.

- A VEP (Visual Evoked Potential) gives some brain reception information related to vision, but is not conclusive due to variability.

- Brain scans and neuro-imaging are of value in determining the cause of some symptoms and to rule out some concerns.

- Because CVI cannot always be diagnosed through tests and scans, behavioral characteristics of apparent visual function of children with CVI also contribute significantly to the diagnosis.[14]

After the Diagnosis

Once your child has been diagnosed with CVI, it can be a huge relief. Then intervention can begin. Most parents may feel overwhelmed and daunted at first like we were. You ask yourself what exactly you should be doing and how you will do it all. You wonder if your child will ever be able to see properly. Is there more you can do? Like us, you might want to rush the educational activities because you feel like you are losing precious time. The best thing you can do is to learn as much information as you can about CVI. We hope this book, our website, and the many resources we provide will help you in that goal.

In the next chapter we will discuss the fundamentals of vision and how the eyes and brain work together. We will explore the importance of vision in development so that you can understand why intervention is so important.

4

Vision . . . the Gateway
to the World?

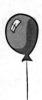

*Although we have the idea that we see things as they really are, in
fact our brain is using shortcuts, best guesses and assumptions
about the world to make our perceptions seem continuous.*

Lea Hyvärinen, MD

Vision, the way the eyes and brain work together to allow us to
see objects and make sense of them, is a deeply personal matter.
We can only see life through our own eyes.

How children interact with the world, and the objects within it, is
largely determined by their visual development. If development
occurs along expected milestones, the way the child sees the
world is likely to be consistent with those around him. However,
challenges in the development of vision can have a profound
effect on the child's self-image, learning, socialization, and other
critical factors in childhood.

This is why it is so important to identify and intervene if there are any problems in visual development. If vision is the gateway to the world, early intervention is the key to unlock the gate.

Visual Development

Let us review how your child's brain develops the ability to process visual information. Research shows that even before the photorecep- tors on the retina are developed in a fetus, the brain starts to form the wiring that will eventually receive the messages from the eyes.[15]

Because the visual system is immature at birth, the first few months after birth represent a critical developmental period in the ability to see well later in life. The optic nerves grow and the visual cortex develops over the first two years of life.[16] The fovia, the area of the retina with cones that allow the eye to see color, and rods that allow the eye to see black and white, comes into maturity around four years of age.

According to the American Optometric Association (AOA),[17] babies at birth are not able to see as clearly as they will when they are older chil- dren or adults. Here are some of the developmental milestones the AOA highlights:

Birth to Four Months

- When babies are born, they tend to focus on objects that have high contrast (meaning light next to dark). Babies cannot yet move their eyes back and forth between two visual targets, and instead focus on objects that are eight to ten inches from their face. This is usually how close a parent holds the baby, and babies are hard- wired to look mostly at their parents in order to bond.

- Within the first few months of life, the eyes start working together and vision improves quickly. This leads to improved hand/eye coordina- tion and the baby can reach out and grasp an object that she sees.

- For the first several months, babies tend to look cross-eyed. This is normal, but if a parent is concerned, an eye evaluation may answer any questions a parent has.

- By three months old, babies are able to follow moving objects with their eyes.

Five to Eight Months

- Hand/eye coordination continues to improve during this period.

- By five months, babies sense depth perception (the ability to tell if an object is nearer or farther away from another object).

- It is generally recognized that babies can see colors by this age range.

- Many babies start crawling during this period, which helps improve hand/eye coordination. Interestingly, babies who learn to walk early and do not crawl for very long may not learn to use their eyes together as well as babies who crawl a lot.

Nine to Twelve Months

- By nine months old, most babies are pulling themselves up to a standing position. Soon after, they are able to use the pincer grasp, which is grasping objects with the thumb and forefinger.

- Babies can now judge distances fairly well.

One to Two Years Old

- By two years of age, most children have well-developed hand/eye coordination.

- This age also shows children using their vision to explore their environment, recognizing familiar objects in picture books, and using a crayon or a pencil to scribble.

When parents are aware of these milestones, they can notice if there are delays in visual development.

How the Eyes and Brain Work Together

In order to identify any problems with visual development in your child, it is necessary to learn how the ability to see develops.

The eyes are among the smallest organs in the body, and yet they play a vital part in processing information. Our eyes work with our brains to tell us how close an object is to us, or where we are in relation to everything around us. The brain and eyes work together to tell us how heavy or light something appears to be, whether it is textured or smooth, and what color and shape it is. When the brain and eyes work together in synchrony, this information is processed within a millisecond.

To understand how the eyes and brain synch together, it's important to look at the structure of the eye and the part of the brain that interacts with the eyes. Here is a simple diagram of the eye.

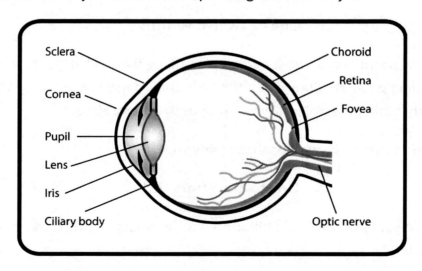

The part of the eye that most people see first is the **iris**. When your baby was born, it was probably one of the first things you looked to see. "What color are her eyes?" This is the part of the eye that is blue, green, brown, or hazel. The iris is very sensitive to light.

Right in the middle of the eyeball is the **pupil,** which is an opening that allows light and visual information into the eye. The iris controls the opening of the pupil. Covering the front of the eyeball is the **cornea,** which is a clear structure. In the back of the front part of the eyeball is the **lens.** The cornea and lens work together to send light images to the back of the eye. The shape of the lens changes depending on whether the eye is looking at something close or far away.

In the back of the eye is a layer of nerve cells called the **retina,** which receives the pictures formed by light rays, and transmits them to the brain through the optic nerve. One area of the retina is called the **fovia,** and it has the highest number of cones that allow the eye to see color and rods that allow the eye to see black and white.

In summary, information is transported from the nerve cells in the retina through the **optic nerve** into the **visual cortex** area of the brain.

An interesting fact about the eyes is that when they bring the image into the brain, the image is reversed—like a camera lens. Here is an image that shows how that happens.

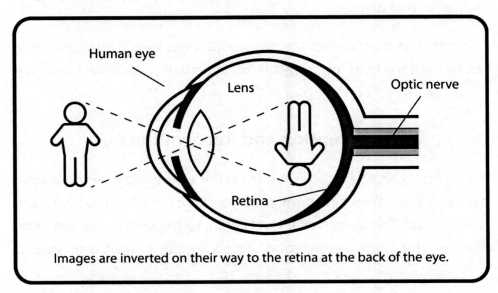

Images are inverted on their way to the retina at the back of the eye.

When your child is looking at an ice cream cone, for example, the image is turned upside down as it goes into the eye. The brain then turns the image right side up and processes the image.

A fact sheet presented by the Blind Babies Foundation mentions the following steps that are involved as the eye sends information to the brain.

• Light rays enter the eye through the cornea; the rays go through the aqueous (the clear watery fluid in front of the lens), the lens, the vitreous (the jelly-like center of the eyeball), and then they hit the rods and cones in the retina.

• The light causes chemical changes in the cells, which then produce electrical activity, similar to how a solar panel can convert light energy to electricity.

• The electrical messages are then sent through the optic nerve to the visual cortex of the brain.

• The visual cortex makes sense of the electrical impulses. It either sends the information to the memory part of the brain or sends a message to the motor area of the brain to tell the body to take some kind of action.

This last step is important for families affected by CVI. The issue may not be with the eyes, but how the brain actually processes the image it is receiving.

Reception and Recognition

We understand how images get from the eye to the brain, but what happens once they get there, and how does the brain understand what it sees? The term "reception" refers to the brain receiving information. The term "recognition" refers to the brain being able to identify an object or behavior as something familiar or unfamiliar.

Researchers have found that, when we look at an object, the eyes move and fixate on the most informative parts of the image.[18] So, if you're looking at a face, the most informative areas are the eyes, the nose, and the mouth. If you are looking at a tree, the most informative parts are the trunk, the branches and the leaves. Your eyes then take a "picture" of that image and send it to the brain.

Next, the visual cortex of the brain forms an internal representation of the image and sends it to the memory area, as if to say, "Hey, have we seen one of these before?" If the memory sends back a "no" response, then the eyes look at more visual information to determine whether or not the motor system needs to get involved. "Is this something to run away from?"

An object is "recognized" if the memory part of the brain can predict how the object will react to certain actions. If you were looking at a face, you would be able to predict how it will move and how it will look while doing certain things. If you are looking at a tree, you can expect it to blow in the wind and leaves to drop from the branches. If the object behaves in unexpected ways, the brain will not recognize it (a face or a tree won't melt, for example).

Children with CVI have a preference for looking at familiar objects, which may tell us something about where in the brain the dysfunction occurs. You might have noticed that your child has an easier time looking at objects that he has seen before.

Spatial Orientation

Another area affected by the ability of the eyes and the brain to communicate is spatial orientation. This is how your child understands where her body is in relationship to the environment. When you think about how complicated the simple act of walking is, you understand how important vision is to spatial orientation. Let's say your child wants to get up from the table and walk into the living room. In order to do this, his eyes must identify the static objects—the chair, the table, the couch in the living room. He then has to use his eyes to see where his body is and activate the motor area of the brain to push the chair away and stand up. Now, his body is in a different position, and the eyes have to adjust to the fact that he is now standing.

As your child walks to the living room, the information coming into his eyes is constantly changing. Things appear to be moving and his body moves in space. The brain is constantly processing the new information as he walks from one room to another. Any disruption in the processing of this "real-time" information can have dramatic consequences in the development of the child.

Visual Reflexes

Visual reflexes can also be affected by disruption in communication between the eyes and the brain. The visual pathways in the brain include a reflexive system and higher levels of visual function. The reflexive level includes a subconscious warning system that alerts a person to take action like using hands to protect the face, avoiding a hazard, or blinking reflexes to close the eyes. Children with CVI often have impaired blink reflexes. The higher visual functions involve memory, language, and spatial orientation, to name a few.

Visual Fields

Another important concept in the understanding of vision is that of visual fields. The visual field is the area of space where all objects are visible simultaneously. In other words, it is what you can see when both of your eyes are open and you are looking straight ahead. It includes peripheral vision, what you can see off to the side.

Your optometrist might have tested this on you by having you look into some goggles and press a button when you saw a light flash to one side or the other of your eyes. In a child, however, the doctor will usually do what is called a "confrontational test." The doctor will sit facing your child and observe the eyes and head to see how much the child can see in the visual field since children may not be able to tell the doctor what they are seeing in their visual field.

One of the reasons that doctors test the visual field is that problems in the visual field can indicate a disease or a disorder of the pathway from the eye to the brain. Visual field problems are common in children with CVI.[19]

Vision's Role in Learning

Vision is a function that serves as a foundation for integrating motor skills and recognition. Motor skills include eye-hand coordination, reaching and grasping, and manual coordination to put an object or food into the mouth. Vision is also believed to be a motivator that triggers larger motor skills like raising the head, rolling over, pushing up, back or forward, and crawling, cruising and eventually walking.

Vision is a necessary skill for recognizing an object and understanding where the object is in space in relation to self. Visual recognition skills include facial recognition, and reading of facial cues and emotions, the skills that support relational skills. Vision triggers a curiosity to explore and learn, which is why interventions for CVI focus on training the brain to see, respond, be curious, and look again for the familiar to build new neural pathways.

Visual Pathways and Brain Injury

Parents, educators, therapists and other professionals who watch how a child with cortical visual impairment functions might not understand why the behaviors they observe are occurring. Yet, this knowledge helps us plan how to modify a child's environment and also determine a child's progress. In addition, we can learn to provide activities appropriate for strengthening those pathways based upon the concept of brain neuroplasticity; that is, the ability of the brain to repair itself and create and strengthen new neural pathways through repetitive learning.

Young children's visual impairments fall into two types.

1. **Ocular impairment** refers to damage to the eye structures through which children receive unclear, limited or no visual information.

2. In **cortical visual impairment**, the ocular structures are healthy, but injury to the visual pathways in the brain prevents a child from interpreting the information that the eyes receive.

Children can have co-existing ocular and cortical impairments.[20]

Dr. Gordon Dutton of Tennent Institute of Ophthalmology and The Royal Hospital for Sick Children of Glasgow, Scotland, has researched, written and published his findings on children with CVI for decades. His writings help us to understand the two visual pathways, their functions, and what happens when an area of that pathway is injured. He kindly shared his writings for this book, and we appreciate his contribution greatly.

Dr. Dutton states that cortical visual impairment "in children includes impaired recognition of people, shapes and objects, and problems with orientation (when the temporal lobes or their connecting pathways are damaged), and difficulty handling complex visual imagery and problems making visually guided movement of the limbs (when the posterior parietal lobes or their connecting pathways are involved).[2]

Part of Dr. Dutton's work has been to describe the functions and the impairments of two visual pathways or streams in the brain. Note the reverse nature of these two visual systems.

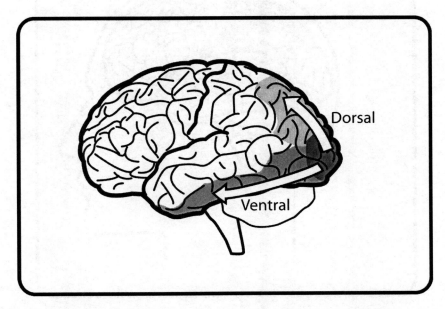

1. The **dorsal pathway** is located between the occipital lobes and the parietal lobes. This system delivers sensory information (sight, smell, sound, taste, and touch) from the external world to the brain. This higher visual pathway, most easily remembered as the WHERE pathway, serves a person's ability to see and process the whole visual scene and carry out visually guided movements. For example, when a child looks down to see steps, assesses if they are steep, and then visually monitors the motion as his feet feel the stairs, he is using his dorsal system.

2. The **ventral system** runs between the occipital lobes and temporal lobe tissue, and its role is to transmit via nerve impulses the interpreted sensory information to the musculoskeletal system in order to execute a proper movement. The ventral system is also called the WHAT pathway because it is involved with object identification, visual recognition and memory.

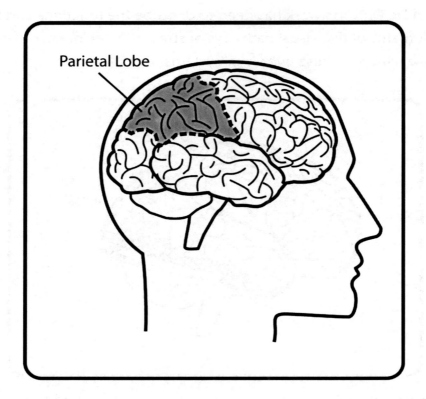

The dorsal stream runs through the parietal cortex. Loss of information to this area of the brain can cause issues in spatial awareness. For example:

• People can see a single element without awareness of the element being part of a larger group or scene. An example is seeing the tree and not the forest or seeing a character on stage but not the surrounding props and scenery.

• Optic ataxia is the absence of using vision to guide arm movements. One example would be a child with CVI who sees a bright red balloon or ball and can recognize the object in space, but when they reach for the ball or balloon, they miss the correct direction and fail to grasp or pick up the object.

• Hemispatial neglect is the condition of being unaware of half of the visual space and focusing on either the right visual field or the left visual field where they can perceive objects. Children with CVI typically have impairment in their lower visual field.

• Inability to perceive motion, which could include not seeing a red balloon passing slowly in front of the face or not seeing the motion of a person walking through a room.

Through the ventral system, one recognizes faces, shapes, objects, and routes by matching incoming data with the brain's library of images. A disorder of the ventral system is called visual agnosia, which means people do not recognize objects. Neither would a person be able to draw or recreate a copy of the object. Knowing the specific area of brain injury can help you understand how to present guidance and create activities to help the brain learn to compensate.

Clearly, the development of vision happens within a narrow window of time in the child's life. If there are problems, it is critical that we intervene and help children learn to create correct images in the brain. With CVI, it is not as simple as getting glasses to correct vision problems in the eyes. This is about helping the child's brain develop the neuronal pathways for vision. While early intervention is best, it is never too late to intervene.

We will present more information about the concept of neuroplasticity, the ability of the brain to restructure itself, in chapter 8. Basically, in learning or practicing a skill, like focusing on a bright pink object, all the neurons in the specific brain area become active at the same time in responding to the stimulation. The neuronal connections become stronger as the neurons fire together; thus repeated exposure to stimuli that our children can easily see creates those neuronal connections. This is how we can teach our children with CVI to learn to see. Next you will read about the Champines and their journey helping their son, Carson, to learn to see.

5
The Champines—
A Diagnosis of CVI

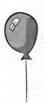

At one glance, I love you with a thousand hearts.
Mihri Hatun

The Champines' First Months

During Kevin and Alicia's pregnancy, they found out from the ultrasound at 20 weeks that they would have a son, and everything seemed fine. Seven weeks later, the circumstances radically changed. Alicia had ultrasounds regularly because of gestational diabetes. At twenty-seven weeks, they found that Carson had hydrocephalus and needed MRIs, which showed that he had pretty severe brain injuries. The doctors did not expect him to live.

The day he was born was an extremely stressful day for everybody. Carson came out breathing independently and started to eat, which was great. After a week in the NICU, the doctors decided that they did not expect Carson to live very long due to low respiration rates and his inability to expel carbon dioxide well. Along with his breathing issues, his MRI scan once again confirmed the severe brain injuries he sustained in utero, which led the neonatologist to believe that Carson's life expectancy would be very short.

Alicia lived at the hospital for the weeks that Carson was there. The point came when the hospice nurse and Carson's doctor met with them to discuss what measures to take if Carson started to decline or stopped breathing. There were times of overwhelming desperation, but there were other times that Kevin and Alicia enjoyed loving on him and playing with him. The family wanted to enjoy the time they had together and see Carson and his seventeen-month old sister, Adrianna, interact.

Yet, time passed, and Carson kept growing and getting stronger.

Alicia shares, "In the very beginning, I struggled because I knew that he had physical delays with his vision. I was so wrapped up in how to best help him. What can I do to give him the absolute best start so that we can build from here? Luckily, an amazing hospice nurse and an amazing therapist both stressed the most important thing I could do is love on him. The most important thing I could do with him is put him in his little bouncer chair and get face to face and talk to him and tickle him and love on him. Thankfully, we were able to breast feed. He did not have any problems with feeding."

"Being able to breast feed Carson, talk and connect with him, take time to be in the rocking chair and not worry about the appropriate toy for his vision were my bonding moments. I was thankful that in my circle at the time, I had people who said, 'The most important thing that you can do is bond with him.' Everything else can come later, but bonding is so important for any newborn, but especially a newborn who does not use his senses fully the way that another typical child would."

Getting a Diagnosis

Over time, Carson continued to thrive. The family's hospice nurse visited weekly after Carson came home and was ecstatic to see how well he was doing. At that point, the family decided to move ahead with meeting with different specialists and getting care and therapy for Carson. The physical therapist was the first to work with Carson.

Alicia continues, "At that time, we knew that he was not using his eyes the way that we remembered our daughter did when she was a newborn. Carson has nystagmus, a type of involuntary eye movement. His eyes always bobbled up and down and side to side. He never looked at us. If we put something close to his face, his eyes never fixated on it. We could tell within the first few weeks that his eyes were not working well. Our physical therapist could tell pretty quickly that he was not responding when she put a red ball and a few other high contrast items in front of his face."

Alicia took two-month-old Carson to Seattle Children's Hospital, the local children's hospital. Moving through three different clinics while there, one of those was with a pediatric ophthalmologist. She did a thorough eye exam with him, dilated his eyes, and made sure his eyes looked okay. From that, she found that his optic nerves were pale. The Champines later learned that a normal optic nerve looks pink, almost a red color, meaning there is a lot of blood flow. Carson's optic nerves were pale, which means there was not a lot of blood flow going through because of the brain injuries. The worst of Carson's brain injuries are on the right side of his brain, in the middle and towards the back. Some areas were so damaged by the brain hemorrhages he suffered that there is no longer brain tissue. Fluid fills a lot of that area now.

The ophthalmologist looked at Carson's MRI and said that his vision was probably affected because there was damage where the visual pathways are in the brain. After looking at the MRI and doing tests to see how he responded to different visual stimuli, and then doing a thorough eye check, she gave the official diagnosis that he had cortical visual impairment.

Learning How to Help

Alicia continues with the story: "We immediately contacted our family support person at the Birth to Three program and told her that we had gotten the official diagnosis. She got us in touch with a teacher of the visually impaired and we were connected with our TVI, Diane. We were very lucky that we started working with a teacher of the visually impaired so early."

"That part of being mom, like I did with my typical daughter, is core. I'm thankful that I started off that way because I think, as Carson has gotten older, our routines have helped. Like in the morning, typically, we get up; we do diaper change and change our clothes. During that time, I talk with him and love him. But also during that time, I do leg stretches with him. So Carson thinks we are playing and communicating on his changing table, but I am also stretching his legs. Our teacher of the visually impaired suggested we have a visual element that is always there at each station in the house so that Carson will see a consistent visual and will recognize he is on the changing table."

"While on the changing table, he always looks to the left, up on his wall, where we put a bunch of CDs. We turned them and pasted them against the wall so the shiny, reflective part faces outward. Carson got very excited about those. We love it because now when I do a diaper change, it is a time for us to talk and me to tickle him. But it is also a place where he is able to use his vision to see his CDs that he loves on the wall."

The Champines learned that kids with CVI might struggle to use their vision if they are simultaneously trying to do anything else. So if you have a child who does not have a lot of muscle control or strength in their neck and back, their vision may shut down from fatigue if they are also trying to use those muscles. If you put them in a physical position where they have to work hard keeping their body steady, they may have a harder time using their vision because they can only handle one sensory thing at a time.

When working with Carson on vision tasks, they placed Carson in a very comfortable position. For him, it was usually lying on his back, where he did not have to use his neck and back muscles. He could fully concentrate on whatever it is they had put in front of him to see.

The vision therapist also taught the Champines to make things easy to see for Carson, meaning to have one object, not a bunch of different ones. Alicia explains: "Right now, I am in my living room, sitting here and I am looking at my hand. I can also see behind it my television, my daughter's toys, my son's stander, and a red balloon. If I had CVI, I would see the hand in front of me as blended in with everything else in the background. We needed to make the background for him blank and plain. So we bought tri-fold boards that people use at science fairs. Whatever we show Carson is placed in front of the board to cut out all the clutter of the background."

"At Christmas time, Carson responded to a bright orange octopus, and we realized he was actually responding to something visually. We started using bright orange in a lot of different toys, such as a bright orange helicopter. To work with Carson, we made sure he was lying on the floor so he was not using his body for support. We put that one object in front of him and then we would put a black background behind it, and he could fully concentrate on looking at that one object."

"Diane was the person who gave me these basic rules of how to help Carson use his vision. I also am a huge researcher, so I did research on the Internet, checking out forums and different groups where parents share ideas and ask questions. I quickly connected with other parents who had children with CVI. I think that was one of the biggest resources for me—talking to other parents that have been there. I am on Facebook a lot so I found a few groups on Facebook for people with CVI or who have children with CVI. I found Yahoo! had a group that was for CVI. Through that, I learned ideas of what things kids respond to like shiny, shimmery Mardi Gras necklaces or beads. I loved that idea because Carson would reach out and try to touch them. He liked the tactile feel in his hands, plus he was able to see them if we placed them in front of him with a blank background."

"Connecting with other parents and hearing what worked for them was how I learned the basic stuff that you could do at home. You can read a lot about the theory behind CVI, but we needed to know what to do in our daily lives. How do we apply something for Carson throughout the day? Parents were the key for me in learning different strategies to use."

"In the very beginning, Carson only wanted to respond to reflective type things. I purchased a reflector-type sun visor that you put in your car and cover the windshield to keep the heat out. Carson loved the foil reflection, and it was the one place where he would do tummy time, and he would be content because of the reflection. In the very beginning, Carson needed the shiny Mardi Gras beads, mirrors, and reflective objects."

Now, Alicia can put toys in front of him that are not shiny. They are a matte finish and brightly colored. He responds to those. While on the floor, Alicia would lay an item in front of him and he would reach out and touch it. Some of his toys make noise, and he knows that that is a certain toy. Alicia also pointed out that they use consistent, familiar toys with Carson. Carson has about ten toys total that the family uses on a regular basis because children with cortical visual impairment like repetition. They like things that are constant and familiar.

Alicia shares: "With my daughter, who has perfect vision, we can put out any toy and she would respond to and be excited about it. But Carson needs that consistency to be able to use his vision on that toy. He loves his iPad. My husband bought him an iPad about six months ago to use. Carson also has a stander that he uses because he does not bear weight in his legs. He has a stander that we put him in twice a day. During that time, we also put the iPad out and that is where he can start interacting with the iPad. We turn down all the lights in the room. We try to minimize the sounds. Obviously, I have an almost three-year-old, so she is very loud. But he has gotten pretty used to his sister's loudness. We try to keep the sound down a little bit so he can concentrate on looking at the iPad, using his hand to make things, make noise on the iPad or change colors."

"So that is how we start the day. We have times where he is sitting in his chair or on the floor, and my daughter and I are playing and we hand him some toys and have playtime together. For us, it does not work to set aside two hours every day that we are going to devote to therapy. With having another child, my schedule does not allow for that. We find that it is pretty easy throughout the day to stretch Carson's legs or put him in his stander, or do tummy time, or use our iPad."

In fact, it turns out that this is better for children with CVI. Incorporating opportunities to use vision throughout the day is far more effective than setting aside an hour or two just for vision.

"Our daughter does not remember life before Carson because she was so young when he was born. She is always very caring for him. She will hand him toys. If he were crying and upset, she would say 'Mom, why is Arson crying?' (She calls him Arson instead of Carson). Or she would go to get his binky. If we are getting ready to go somewhere, she asks if Carson is coming, too. Typically, in the morning, I get her out of bed first. We then go and get her brother. She usually wants him to see whatever toy she is playing with. We put it in front of him to see and she also puts it close to his hand so that he can feel it. It is amazing how she already knows that he 'sees things' with his hands as much as his eyes."

"She does not want to play yet with him. I think he is still not able to move around and be mobile yet, and she is doing her thing. So she does not necessarily interact with him during playtime. But throughout the day, she is very caring and wants to know where he is. She is always careful with him. Recently, I have started leaving the two of them in a room while I step out. I will say, 'You take care of your brother. Make sure he's okay?' She agrees. So now she is being his little mommy when I am out of the room."

"It is fun to be able to watch those sorts of interactions. There are times when she gets annoyed with him like I think any sibling would, especially if she wants to use the iPad, but it is his visual time in his stander. She would ask, 'Why does Arson get the iPad?' Aside from typical sibling stuff, she seems to love him and care for him. That is one blessing of having them so close together."

Alicia's story of Carson's needs is very similar to events that engulfed our family in bringing Lukas home from the hospital and learning to adapt to varied therapies. Many children with CVI have other physical challenges as well as having CVI. While it's important to start vision therapy early, it is also important to start any other necessary therapies as early as possible to help your child develop during the critical years of brain development.

In the United States, young children with CVI are eligible to receive these therapies through Early Intervention Programs (EIP) through their city, county or state agencies. Each EIP defines its eligibility requirements and services offered on a local basis, although the national U.S. law provides guidelines, all of which are covered in chapter 11.

Now that you have an idea of how vision works, what CVI is, how it can be diagnosed, how families adapt, and what services can be provided, let's discuss the characteristics of CVI in more depth so you can begin to piece together a plan for helping your own child learn to see.

6
Characteristics of CVI

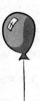

Anyone can give up; it's the easiest thing in the world to do.
But to hold it together when everyone else would understand
if you fell apart, that's true strength.
Christopher Reeves

Two Sets of Traits

Due to inaccurate perceptions or a lack of knowledge about children with CVI, only in the last two decades have we seen professionals identify traits of children with CVI. These traits fall into two categories: the physical presentation of the eyes and the behavioral traits that a parent, teacher, or medical doctor can observe over time. We touched on these in chapter 3, but we will expand on them in more depth here.

Presentation of the Eyes

As mentioned earlier, children with cortical visual impairment typically do not look blind. As a result of their impaired vision, however, they may have a blank facial expression, a lack of visual communication skills and eye movements that appear smooth, but don't seem to really focus on anything. Children with CVI may also demonstrate the following physical traits:

Strabismus is the medical term for eye turning, often nicknamed by the public as crossed-eyes, wandering-eye, or deviating eye. The condition of strabismus occurs periodically if stress or illness causes the deviation. Parents of children with CVI are more likely to see a consistent eye turning or deviation when a child looks at an object. Eye doctors look for strabismus when one looks at an object twenty feet away or close up at thirteen inches for a child, in both side-to-side and up-down directions. Please note **intermittent strabismus** is a normal developmental milestone for children up to six months of age. After six months, it needs to be evaluated.

For children with CVI, strabismus could be an early sign, especially if consistent exotropia is present.[22] **Exotropia** is a common type of strabismus, in which the eye turns away from the nose, called outward deviation, and occurs consistently when a child is looking at either near or distant objects.

Children with CVI could also display a slight **motor nystagmus**, an unsteady gaze or jerky eye movements. This would be a result of injured cortical control.

Another condition called **sensory nystagmus** is an easy-to-see unsteady eye fixation. Children with CVI rarely have this with one exception. "…Unless CVI resides concurrently with another ocular impairment. Likewise, eye pressing, head shaking, and eccentric viewing strategies should NOT be noted in students with cortical visual impairment unless CVI is co-existing with ocular disabilities."[23]

Behavioral Presentations

Professionals working within the field of CVI have documented that children with CVI present similar symptoms. The chart, checklist and discussion of the following characteristics have helped many parents to recognize the presence of CVI in their children. As mom to a daughter with CVI, Krista Williams said, "I did my homework, and when I saw this checklist online, I knew that CVI was exactly what my daughter had. When I took it to her pediatrician the next morning, she agreed. It felt good to finally have a diagnosis. Then I knew my next steps."

Dr. Roman-Lantzy divides CVI into three phases. Most children start in Phase I, which means that most of the CVI characteristics are present. As a child progresses through the three phases, many of the characteristics begin to resolve. This process can take several years and requires diligence and persistence. Children in Phase III approach near normal vision to varying degrees and may even be able to attain literacy. Her CVI Resolution Chart, on the following pages, outlines the basic characteristics of CVI and shows how they typically resolve as a child moves through the three phases.

CVI Characteristics	Phase I Building Visual Behavior Level I Environmental Considerations		Phase II Integrating Vision with Function Level II Environmental Considerations		Phase III Resolution of CVI Characteristics Level III Environmental Considerations
	Range 1-2 (0)	Range 3-4 (.25)	Range 5-6 (.50)	Range 7-8 (.75)	Range 9-10 (1)
Color preference	Objects viewed are generally single color	Has favorite color	Objects may have 2-3 favored colors	More colors, familiar patterns regarded	No color or pattern preferences
Need for movement	Objects viewed generally have movement/ reflective properties	More consistent localization, brief fixations on movement and reflective materials	Movement continues to be an important factor to initiate visual attention	Movement not required for attention at near	Typical responses to moving targets
Visual latency	Prolonged periods of visual latency	Latency slightly decreases after periods of consistent viewing	Latency present only when student is tired, stressed, or overstimulated	Latency rarely present	Latency resolved
Visual field preferences	Distinct field dependency	Shows visual field preferences	Field preferences decreasing with familiar inputs	May alternate use of right and left fields	Visual fields unrestricted
Difficulties with visual complexity	Responds only in strictly controlled environments Generally, no regard of the human face	Visually fixates when environment is controlled	Student tolerates low levels of familiar background noise Regards familiar faces when voice does not compete	Competing auditory stimuli tolerated during periods of viewing; student may now maintain visual attention on musical toys Views simple books or symbols Smiles at/regards familiar and new faces	Only the most complex visual environments affect visual response Views books or other two-dimensional materials. Typical visual/social responses

| CVI Characteristics | Phase I — Building Visual Behavior | | Phase II — Integrating Vision with Function | | Phase III — Resolution of CVI Characteristics |
| | Level I Environmental Considerations | | Level II Environmental Considerations | | Level III Environmental Considerations |
	Range 1-2 (0)	Range 3-4 (.25)	Range 5-6 (.50)	Range 7-8 (.75)	Range 9-10 (1)
Light-gazing and nonpurposeful gaze	May localize briefly, but no prolonged fixations on objects or faces Overly attentive to lights or perhaps ceiling fans	Less attracted to lights; can be redirected to other targets	Light is no longer a distracter		
Difficulty with distance viewing	Visually attends in near space only	Occasional visual attention to familiar, moving, or large targets at 2-3 feet	Visual attention extends beyond near space, up to 4-6 feet	Visual attention extends to 10 feet with targets that produce movement	Visual attention extends beyond 20 feet Demonstrates memory of visual events
Atypical visual reflexes	No blink in response to touch and/or visual threat	Blinks in response to touch, but response may be latent	Blink response to touch consistently present Visual threat response intermittently present	Visual threat response consistently present (both reflexes near 90% resolved]	Visual reflexes always present; resolved
Difficulty with visual novelty	Only favorite or known objects elicit visual attention	May tolerate novel objects if the novel objects share characteristics of familiar objects	Use of "known" objects to initiate looking sequence	Selection of objects less restricted, 1-2 sessions of "warm up" time required	Selection of objects not restricted
Absence of visually guided reach	Look and touch occur as separate functions Look and touch occur with large and/or moving objects	Look and touch occur with smaller objects that are familiar, lighted, or reflective Look and touch are still separate	Visually guided reach used with familiar objects or "favorite" color	Look and touch occur in rapid sequence, but not always together	Look and touch occur together consistently

Key

- Draw an X through boxes that represent resolved visual behaviors
- Use highlighter to outline boxes describing current visual functioning
- Draw an O in boxes describing visual skills that may never resolve because of coexisting ocular conditions

Reprinted with permission of author Christine Roman-Lantzy and the publisher American Foundation for the Blind

The following behavioral presentations are adapted from the 2010 version of Dr. Roman-Lantzy's *Cortical Visual Impairment* and cited research sources. With each of the following characteristics, it is important to remember that it will often resolve as your child's vision improves through intervention.

1. Color Preference is commonly seen in children with CVI. These children have color perception, which is thought to be less susceptible to elimination because both the left and the right sides of the brain perceive color, and the perceptual areas may be more protected from oxygen deprivation and injury.

Infants without brain injury see colors at one week after birth. They first see red, orange, yellow and green, but it takes a little longer for them to see blue and violet colors, which have shorter wavelengths. Fewer color receptors exist in the human retina for blue light.

Children with CVI often have a preferred color, particularly in the early phases. Red and yellow tend to be the most common preferred colors probably because they have the longest wavelengths and the human eye has more receptors for long wavelengths. Some children may prefer other colors, such as bright orange or pink, or even enjoy seeing shiny or mirrored objects. Whether or not a child is able to name colors is a function of intact visual memory pathways. Ability to see color can be used to your child's advantage by color-coding objects that might be hard to identify otherwise.

If you don't know what your child's preferred color is, start by trying objects that are one color and either bright red or bright yellow. By showing Lukas a bright red Elmo doll, we discovered that red was a great color for him early on. As his vision has improved, we have experimented with other colors and found that he now looks at those as well. Once you find a preferred color or colors, place objects with this color throughout your child's day. Try to incorporate it into as many aspects of the daily routine as possible. The more chances your child has to use his vision, the faster vision will improve.

2. Preference for Movement refers to the fact that many children with CVI can see moving objects more easily. Movement enables a child with CVI to gain and keep visual attention. Many children with CVI can locate and track movement as well as maintain their attention on a moving object like a ceiling fan for progressively longer periods. In order to gain and practice visual attention, present material that moves. You might move an object, such as a solid colored stuffed animal back and forth laterally and slowly in front of your child's eyes. Many children with CVI enjoy shiny or reflective objects because they mimic movement. You can build movement for a child into the family's routine and enable children to attend to movement with the use of a mobile, television, certain iPad apps, balloons or reflective objects like CDs. For example, one dad we know of put flat silver balloons on the wall next to his daughter's changing table to catch her attention and encourage her to reach for them.

Given that visual stimulation is very important, Dr. Roman-Lantzy shares in her book *Cortical Visual Assessment* that children will often move their head or body in order to find visual stimulation. Be creative in determining how you position your child and create stimulation for him.[24] For example, another father attached a state flag on his balcony, and his son watched it blow in the wind through the sliding glass door.

3. Latency refers to slow visual responses in two ways: how often or how frequently a child with CVI sees and for what duration. There may be a lag time before the child responds to a visual object like an Elmo doll or bright red balloon. Be patient.

When you present an object, be sure to give the child enough time to respond before taking the object away. Repeat the presentation often for short periods, but consistently over time. After presenting the object, put the Elmo doll in the child's crib. Place the red balloon on a chair at mealtime. Presentation over time familiarizes the child with the color and/or object. Placement of the object in a permanent space encourages visual attention. Also, you can then generalize the familiar color to familiar routines in the child's day.

4. Visual Field Preference refers to the fact that almost all children with CVI have preferences in their visual field; that is, where they are best able to see and attend. Close observation by parents and therapists will determine how to assist the child in training the brain to see. For example, a child may not attend to an object presented directly in front of them, but will look if the item is placed on one side or another or will turn their head to view the object. Many children with CVI find it easiest to use their peripheral vision. This may be because the part of the brain that interprets motion and peripheral vision is small and located in the back of the brain on both sides, making it harder to injure. For this reason, movement, especially in the peripheral field, can often trigger a child to begin using their vision.

Another child, however, may be better at seeing items placed in a central location in front of her, and may perhaps also be better at detail or facial recognition. It is important to closely observe your child's head and movement, and noting when she has seen a target. In this way, you can ensure that you always present items in your child's preferred field, increasing her chances of seeing them.

When we show a new object to Little Bear, we typically begin by presenting it to his left side, which is his preferred visual field. With more familiar objects, however, he is able to look at them in other parts of his visual field. Like many children with CVI, Lukas also has trouble viewing items in his lower visual field. As a result, we always make sure items are raised or hanging overhead so that he will be able to see them. This, too, is improving over time.

5. Light-gazing and Nonpurposeful Gazing are very commonly seen in children with CVI. Light-gazing may be observed in roughly 60 percent of all children with CVI.[25] Children with CVI may tend to compulsively stare at light, may be attracted visually to bright lights, or frequently look at a specific light. Light can be used to help attract a child's attention to a visual target. Many TVIs will use light boxes for this reason. Light boxes are offered by the American Printing House for the Blind (APH) and have, "a lighted translucent white work surface, providing a high contrast background for opaque materials and a source of illumination for colored transparent and translucent items."[26]

Your TVI or other vision specialist should be able to help you get a light box and other materials from the American Printing House for the Blind (APH). Any child who is enrolled in a school or Early Intervention Program with a documented visual impairment is eligible for materials from APH. In order to qualify for materials, the child must be registered with APH, which should be done immediately upon enrollment in early intervention or school. Typically, it is a TVI or other vision specialist who registers the child, which then allows APH to offer the materials through the Federal Quota Program. If for some reason a child is not enrolled in either an Early Intervention or school program, their family can contact APH directly. For more information about the Federal Quota Program and APH, you can visit: www.aph.org/fedquotpgm/fedquota.htm.

Although you can purchase a light box directly from the American Printing House for the Blind, they are also often available to borrow from your TVI or other vision specialist.

Nonpurposeful gazing refers to the child not attending to a visual target, seeming to look at something that isn't there or looking at things without intent. No one knows for certain why this behavior is so common in children with CVI. Is the child simply staring? Is the child turning away from overwhelming stimuli? Is she turning away from an object while processing information and making sense of the lesson or the environment?

Paying attention to your child's preferences and behavior can help you better plan visual activities. Ask yourself which actions draw your child's attention. If your child turns away, what seemed to trigger that response? Has fatigue set in? Notice what fatigue looks like and how your child displays fatigue. Team members who assist your child with CVI will also do functional assessments, and your input as a team member is invaluable.

6. Difficulty with Visual Complexity refers to the difficulty for a child with CVI to distinguish complex visual fields. For example, a child may not be able to find a solid colored ball on a multicolored rug, but they would be able to find it if the rug were black. Placing a black background behind an object will make it much easier for your child to see. There are many ways to accomplish this. The American Printing House for the Blind sells Invisiboards, which are forty-eight by thirty inch trifold boards that eliminate visual clutter with a solid white, slick material on one side and a solid black, Velcro compatible material on the other. Parents have come up with other creative ways to reduce visual clutter. For example, you can place a black presentation board behind the object, as Alicia did with Carson, or you can hang a black sheet or pillowcase on the wall behind the object. Many parents have also created "little rooms" for their children out of PVC pipe and black cloth, which help block out competing sensory input. The important thing is to eliminate background complexity so that your child can focus solely on the object you wish him to see.

Similarly, it is also important that the object itself is visually simple. Children in the early phases of CVI may be unable to look at a toy that is more than one or two colors, even if the background is simple. For this reason, it is important to begin with single-colored items. Many children's toys are too complex for children with CVI. Parents often find that the best "toys" for their children actually come from the dollar store or the party store. Some of Lukas' favorite party store toys include red or yellow Mylar balloons, red Mardi Gras beads, and a bright red Valentine's Day cascade centerpiece. Valentine's Day and Christmas are great times of year to keep an eye out for CVI-appropriate items. The American Institute for the Blind also lists fifty toy suggestions for young children, including pom-poms, glass mirror ball ornaments, silver tinsel, gold tinsel, neon tube lights, glitter twist spinners, or solid color cat toys like balls with sound and color which activate when rolled.

The principle of avoiding visual complexity also applies to sensory input, such as a sibling playing nearby or the constant drone of the television, competing for the child's attention in the environment. When presenting a visual item to your child, it may be tempting to carry on a dialogue about the item, but this may actually make it harder for your child to see. Toys that feature too much noise can be just as difficult for children with CVI as those with too many colors. Because it can be difficult for children with CVI to look and listen simultaneously, you may find that your child turns away from you when you talk to him. It is easy to think your child is ignoring you, but in fact, he may be turning away so that he can focus on what you are saying without having to use his vision at the same time. Creating a simple environment is a matter of eliminating noise, visual clutter and anything else that might distract from the visual task.

7. Difficulty in Distance Viewing refers to the fact that children with CVI may only attend in the near space or bring objects near for magnification. This action might also reduce the "crowding" of objects in the background. If the panorama is too complex because the background is highly patterned, there are too many objects or objects are spaced too closely together, there may be difficulty in distance viewing. Your child may be able to see objects further away if they are larger or placed in front of a plain background.

8. Atypical Reflex Responses refers to a child with CVI not responding or responding in delayed fashion when an object like a toy or a hand comes too close to the eyes or touches the bridge of the nose. Because this response can't be taught and it resolves as the other characteristics of CVI resolve, it can be a good quick way to assess a child's progress. When we first began working with Little Bear, we noticed that he often wouldn't blink at all in response to a visual threat. Now, he often blinks, though it is still delayed.

9. Difficulty with Visual Novelty refers to the child with CVI who only looks at familiar or favorite objects, with little regard to new objects. The child does not demonstrate curiosity for novel visual objects.

This is a critical point for parents and professionals to understand, because you may be trained to think that novel experiences are enriching. You typically learn in the early years to help children increase resilience and confidence by trying new things, but this is not true for the child with CVI.

Remember, the familiar is the favorite and K. I. S. S., which stands for "keep it the same and simple." These sayings will remind you that you are training new brain pathways, and the synapses become thicker and stronger when using the same routine consistently for short periods of time. With Lukas, we found that, over time, many of his CVI characteristics disappeared when looking at familiar objects, but are still very much present with new objects. For example, he shows no latency these days when looking at Elmo, but still needs time to respond to an object he's never seen before.

When introducing new objects, a good rule of thumb is to make sure the new object is not dramatically different from the child's familiar objects. If your child responds well to red, shiny Mardi Gras beads, you may want to try yellow Mardi Gras beads or a red, shiny balloon. By changing only one feature of the object, it may still be familiar enough to capture your child's visual attention.

10. Decreased Visually Guided Reach refers to a child reaching out and touching an object without coordination of eye-hand movement. In other words, often a child with CVI will look away from the object and then reach for it. The child does not coordinate looking and reaching so she may look away during the act of reaching. The child may exhibit decreased accurate reaching and sometimes reach for an object better with her eyes closed.

Other Common Characteristics

As mentioned in chapter 3, a few other characteristics are common among children with CVI. You may hear it said that the vision of a child with CVI changes throughout the day. While it often appears this way, in fact it is not the child's vision that changes, but her ability to use her vision that changes. Fatigue, auditory distractions, too much background complexity, or inappropriate positioning can make it much more difficult for a child with CVI to use her vision. The Blind Babies Foundation explains it this way, "When a child with CVI needs to control his head, use his vision, and perform fine motor tasks, the effort can be compared to a neurologically-intact adult learning to knit while walking a tightrope."[27] If your child's vision seems to change, it is worth exploring if any environmental factors are the cause and adjusting these as needed.

Because visual activities are difficult for children with CVI, the child may fatigue easily. This is another reason that incorporating visual activities into the daily routine is preferable to setting aside an hour or two for "vision therapy." Repetition and consistency throughout the day will yield far better results than creating solid blocks of "vision time." In this way, you can also make sure that the visual activities are functional and meaningful. You can teach your child to associate certain items with diaper changing, feeding, bath time and other routines in his day. The use of vision then has a purpose rather than just creating a visual activity out of context.

Remember that, as parents, you have the opportunity to help your child with CVI to expand their visual skills through the brain's ability to form new visual pathways and learn new interactions. This is a promising time in the field of CVI with research, interest, and people of good heart contributing to the pool of shared knowledge amongst parents and professionals. If you follow your child's lead, pay attention to the characteristics she displays and get creative, you will find ways to help your child learn to see!

7

The Thathachari's Journey with CVI

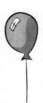

If the wind will not serve, take to the oars.

Latin Proverb

Like many of you on your family journeys with cortical visual impairment, in the maze of doctors, medications, and seeking answers, Geetha and Aravind Thathachari were happy to finally receive a diagnosis for their son well into his first year of life. Many families have found that getting a diagnosis is a relief. Knowing that your child has CVI allows you to begin to take the necessary steps to help your child.

In the Thathachari family journey, they came to a new country and found excellent medical resources for their son. As the mom, Geetha, shares her story, note her emotional honesty as well as the resilience of her words and heart. She describes her son's skill levels and their goals for him.

In the Beginning

Aravind Thathachari and his wife Geetha relocated from India to Orlando, Florida as employees of a tech company in 2007. They had been married close to two and a half years and they had planned to have a baby. Geetha became pregnant, and felt blessed to be healthy as she carried her first born.

On October 29, 2009, Geetha went through twenty-three hours of labor, and their son was born at thirty-eight weeks via cesarean section, as the baby did not descend. They named their son Sripathi, a Hindu name meaning *abode of prosperity*. At delivery, it was determined that he had a large head, which an MRI confirmed. At twenty days he had a head ultrasound, which came back normal. Aravind and Geetha took their son home, and he seemed fine for two months.

On December 29, 2009, Sripathi was given the second month of scheduled vaccines, which were DTaP, Hep B dose 2 and oral Rotavirus. Geetha feels this triggered her son's seizures. He had recurrent seizures and was taken to the emergency room on January 1, 2010. He was on several seizure medications in the next two months, which included Phenobarbital, Keppra, and Topomax. None of the medications could control his seizures. On February 26, 2010, at Texas Children's Hospital, Sripathi was diagnosed with Cryptogenic Localization-Related Epilepsy with tonic versive seizures, and independent left and right hemisphere seizures. Other diagnoses included developmental encephalopathy with global delays, prominent hypotonia, and macrocephaly, all of which suggested a neuro-metabolic disorder.

On March 5th, Sripathi had his MRI and the results stated that his brain had abnormally increased subcortical and periventricular white matter volume with abnormal thickening of the corpus callosum.

On March 9th, Sripathi was scheduled for further blood work to test for markers of Alexander's disease, of Canavan's disease, and amino acid plasma. All of this blood work eventually came back negative except for the chromosomal micro array or CMA. Doctors found that Sripathi has PHF8 gene duplication on the X chromosome. Sripathi also had his eyes checked by a neuro-ophthalmologist and was diagnosed with cortical visual impairment.

Geetha explains, "The neurologist suggested the chromosomal microarray analysis, which tells us if there is a chromosomal error and in which chromosome it might be. The test revealed that Sripathi had a duplicate gene called PHF8 on the X chromosome. The neurologist was able to tell us exactly what seizure he was having, which part of the brain triggers the seizures and what needed to be done to control them. But they could not tell what causes this in him."

"Even in genetics testing, though they found this particular gene is duplicated in the X chromosome, they said they have never seen this anywhere else in the world. Sripathi is the only one. Later, the doctors did blood work on me because it was on the X chromosome, and they found the same gene being duplicated in me, but I turned out fine. The geneticists were suggesting that maybe if it was a girl child, she would not have had so many complications because this gene is probably acting funny for a boy. So we still do not know much about that."

Sripathi, at sixteen months of age, was weaned off Phenobarbital. At about seventeen months, Sripathi started getting infantile spasms. His neurologist prescribed Zonisamide. Sripathi receives physical therapy (PT), occupational therapy (OT), vision therapy (VT), speech therapy (ST) and aqua therapy.

"There was one clue that the doctors had about why he has CVI. Sripathi's head is enlarged because the white matter is growing too much, and it is actually compressing on his cortex, like pressing on his nerves at the back, which affects vision. That could be one of the reasons, but they cannot really say for sure because they have never seen this before."

"Prognosis is very weak at this point. At the rate the white matter is growing, we cannot say if his cognitive skills will catch up. The ophthalmologist told us that his vision, the nerves of his eyes are all perfect. So the brain is not able to understand whatever it is getting. If the white matter is going to keep pressing on his nerves at the back, even though we give intervention, how long it will be able to fight the compression and catch up is unknown."

Making Progress

Geetha shares, "The doctors said when we returned to Orlando from the Texas Children's Hospital in Houston, the first thing to do is talk to Early Steps, an early intervention program in our city, and tell them that we needed vision services. Even the neurologist suggested that we start getting him PT services through early intervention. We found the local intervention coordinator quite supportive. After the visitation and the paperwork, they evaluated Sripathi at the developmental center. Then they referred us to Lighthouse of Central Florida. Initially, they said they will give only PT services, and at seven months, the PT came in. By eighth months the vision therapy was started. She was also supportive to make sure that Sripathi was not too agitated the first time somebody came or touched him. She avoided using perfumes so that the smells did not trigger seizures or trigger an aversion to someone new. She was concerned about Sripathi and was very supportive."

"Back then, I really did not reach out to many people I did not know about CVI. When I talk to many parents now, they say that their vision therapists do not know what CVI is. Therefore, the parents have to teach them so they are able to help with intervention. Our vision therapist had been trained in CVI. She took care of everything, like making sure how we handled him, and she taught me how to introduce him to new situations, which was very helpful."

"By the time we contacted specialists and started therapy, Sripathi was seven months old, but we had already seen a drastic change within two months. When we started therapy, Sripathi was not able to see someone coming into the room unless there was a window open and a shadow passed. Even when my husband or I stood next to him, he was not able to look at us. Within two months of vision therapy, in which the therapist showed Sripathi the light box for forty-five minutes, this made a drastic change. He was able to look at us, and then look at us straight in our face, and when we moved he would follow us. That was an amazing time. That is how we progressed from the initial diagnosis."

Relocating to Texas

Geetha continues, "We relocated to Irving, Texas for my husband's job in March 2011 about the time Sripathi turned seventeen months. The Florida early intervention coordinator transferred Sripathi's records to the early intervention program in Irving. Launch Ability was the service provider and I had to follow up with them for several weeks and they finally came to our home to evaluate Sripathi on May 17, 2011."

"It was worth the wait as all his new therapists were understanding and caring. His PT is very supportive and has guided us in getting Sripathi a standing frame. The OT is encouraging and very caring with Sripathi during therapy. Sripathi likes his developmental therapist because she gives him good massages! In Texas, the school district provides for vision services. So we contacted the school district and Ms. Cynthia was kind enough to come in and evaluate Sripathi during the summer break. She has inspired me with several ideas for vision intervention with Sripathi."

"Now at age two, Sripathi is an adorable boy who loves familiar music and books being read to him. He likes to be engaged in activity though as an extremely passive participant. Due to his cortical visual impairment and severe hypotonia, he has never had the urge to reach, touch, feel and grab things around him. He dislikes and many times would cry hard when we do certain therapy positions, which force him to hold his heavy head (due to macrocephaly) up at midline. In spite of this, he tolerates a few minutes at a time of sitting on a stool with support to his trunk and also wearing his compression garment and orthotics. When left unattended he does not move much and sometimes falls asleep, otherwise he is a very cheerful child."

"He has cortical visual impairment and also has nystagmus. He notices familiar objects like certain pictures on the wall, books, toys, the light box, the mirror, and us, his parents. He has a sensory play area that is covered in black and yellow colors. The area has ribbons and a slinky hanging from above. Sripathi tends to look only upwards for some time and gradually goes to sleep."

"We have found from the past visual therapy in Florida that he showed marked improvement with the use of only a light box and one single toy shown repeatedly. In addition, we need to determine his focal area. So we are able to get his maximum attention during any activity."

"Most evenings after his snack, we help him do some finger painting. He does not see his hands or the paint or the paper while painting. Although he sometimes pulls his hands away while we hold them to paint, at the same time, he does not fuss much. After he is done, we show him the art work and often he gives it a glance."

How to Cope

Geetha explained how she and her husband have different coping skills. She says, "My husband is very strong. He just trusts in God, but

I am a person who keeps questioning everything. I have questioned, found answers and taken courses to educate myself. I used to do all intervention, as I have my own schedule for Sripathi."

"There are times when I am cooking or eating, I get so depressed. My moods happen in intervals when I am not focused on doing my son's interventions. I make sure my frustration or anger or depression is between his interventions, but it is there sometimes. At times, I am fine and I will try my best to take care of things. I will be high one day and then low some days. So it is still back and forth."

"My support for the CVI comes from the Jewish Guild for the Blind's weekly conference calls on which I am quite regular. I get a lot of ideas and suggestions from parents on the call. They have guest speakers and Dr. Roman joins the call once a month, so that is really amazing and has been the best support. Apart from that, the intervention therapists feel that I am one parent who stays with them during the therapy and learns from them. I do my own sets of the interventions with Sripathi. They feel happy about that so they give me more suggestions. My parents have visited from India, and they also help as they can."

"When I started doing therapy and interventions with Sripathi, I noticed that he was interested on some days, and other days, he was not. The therapist indicated this was true for most children with CVI. They fatigue easily. Although Sripathi cannot do much, when I show him certain books and he looks at them, I feel so happy, and I think *Oh my god, he is actually seeing the book,* which encourages me to get similar books. It is nice when I get responses from him, like an acknowledgement when he does something, as it motivates me to do more and more."

"I follow a routine with him. As soon as he wakes up, there will be a set of visual interventions that I do with him. When he is rested, then I do physical interventions with him, like the physical therapist suggested with a medium size ball: rock him back and forth and side to side. During the initial days, he cried a lot when we put him on his stomach on the ball, but now he has learned to lift and somewhat balance his head when placed on the ball on his stomach. He actually enjoys rocking on the ball."

"Next, there will be a routine for his bath. I show him a picture of him in the bathtub saying, 'Okay, this is your bath time. You are going to go take a bath.' Then I give him a massage and put him in the bath. In the tub, when I tell him that I am going to put water on his face now, and I count one, two, three, four. On the count of four, I put the water on his face. On the count of four, he closes his eyes and is ready, anticipating that water is going to go on his face. Those small comprehensions make me feel good, like I have to do more and he will learn on the go. After the bath, I put him on the towel and say, 'Close your eyes, I am going to wipe your face.' There are days he will really close his eyes. Next, I explain, 'I'm going to put some powder on you, and we will brush you and everything.' Brushing gives him sensory input."

"My husband is quite encouraging whenever he finds time. When I do visual interventions, I will put Sripathi on my lap and I will show things in front of him. To understand what Sripathi is learning, I call my husband to sit next to me, watch Sripathi, and tell me what I need to do better so he can concentrate better. In that way, he is very supportive."

Educational Methods

Geetha shares: "I still mainly use Dr. Roman's methods. Recently, my vision therapist gave me the Sensory Learning Kit from APH (The American Printing House for the Blind), along with the assessment, a guide and all the equipment that I can use with him. I just started this in February of 2012. I want to do an assessment every week and compare all the weeks together and understand his progress better."

"In August of 2011, the vision therapist gave me an invitation from the school district to go to the Dallas Museum of Art. We attended an art session with a blind artist named Mr. John Bramblitt. This particular artist also had seizures. At the age of ten, he lost his vision completely due to seizures. He was so frustrated at that time, he asked his mother to buy him some paint and he wanted to do art. Though his mother was skeptical, still she bought it for him. Slowly, he started painting. At the end of the day, when she saw the painting she was amazed that he could do so much. This artist taught me a technique to use fabric paint to draw an outline like of a dog in pencil, then outline the dog image with the fabric paint and let it dry. So the next day I showed it to Sripathi on a light box, made him feel the outline of the dog image and explained this is the shape of a dog, and we started finger painting into the dog."

"I used to do a lot of finger painting with him—just putting paint on his fingers and scribbling and moving. He was not really interested, but he was cooperative with me. After I started doing this method of painting, he would see a little bit and watch. After the whole painting is done, he really looks at his painting. I explain his painting to him, and he stares at his painting. This is one method I learned that we enjoy together."

My Inspirations

Geetha says: "It took me a long time, but now I am able to really say that Sripathi is truly a blessing in my life. I was working on a technical job and I had a very fine life. Everything went fine, but I always felt there was a purpose in my life that was lacking. I needed something more to look forward to every day. Now that I am taking care of Sripathi as his mother, teacher and nurse, it has brought a special purpose and a meaning to my life."

"Recently I started a blog. After I saw what Aubri was doing with , I thought I'd do it in a small way based on the interventions that Sripathi receives. My blog is littleidealog.blogspot.com.

This is a way I can share my ideas and suggestions with other parents and caregivers. We all must support each other, share ideas, and stay inspired to help our children."

8

A Reason for Hope: Neuroplasticity

*There is increasing evidence that enriching the environment
can improve cognitive and motor deficits following
a variety of brain injuries.*[28]

Growing Evidence

The quote at the beginning of this chapter is a profound first statement with important implications for children with CVI. The quote summarizes a conclusion of a study with rats, from which researchers generalized conclusions to the human brain. The objective of the study was to determine if the enriched environment in which the rats were raised influenced cognitive functions of normal rats versus rats subjected to drug-induced epileptic seizures at 20 days after birth. Both the rats in the control group and the rats with induced seizures significantly improved visual-spatial learning as a result of the enriched environment. Following the seizures, the enriched environment continued to enhance cognitive functions and "may be due to the plasticity factor."[29] Providing rich environments is exactly what we, as parents, do for our children. We follow our children's lead and offer the enrichment we have found they are responsive to.

The good news is that researchers in the last two decades have found how incredibly adaptable the human brain is and can be. Neuroplasticity is the brain's ability to re-create itself by forming new neurons. Neurons are nerve cells that transmit information and connect one cell to another, forming new pathways for neural communication and restructuring existing ones to support learning and adaptation. The brain forms new neurons until you die. This is a critical concept in discussing CVI because it explains how the brain can rewire itself to take over function of damaged areas. This is how our children can learn to see! Another critical factor is the ability of the brain cells to communicate with one another, continuing to transmit information.

While the concept of plasticity and synaptic growth is more easily understood in the context of young children's growing brains, what about older children with acquired CVI or adults who suffer brain injury from stroke or accidents? Several researchers have used three-dimensional imaging processes in order to observe neural cell growth in mice, from which they generalize the same to the human brain in this conclusion: "...found a real valid model for real-time analysis of neurite outgrowth and the capacity of the adult nervous system to regenerate after injuries."[30] Imagine being able to watch the brain cells reproduce in real time. Our future is now.

Despite the good news, the authors explain that the models of these brain mechanisms are still based upon non-human (mice) models. Furthermore, in order to discover the best ways to trigger neuroplasticity, extensive research is required, which will hopefully allow us a better understanding of how to modify environments for best results in the early years.

In previous chapters discussing brain injury to the visual pathways, you read how the higher visual pathways, the dorsal system and the ventral system work together. In the past, children who experienced injury to these areas were taught compensatory techniques, but it was not assumed that function could be recovered. Why? The brain was thought to be degenerative, rather than regenerative. If brain tissue or neural pathways were damaged, then it was believed that was the end. However, recent evidence suggests that the brain is plastic, meaning it has the ability to reorganize and reconstruct after damage! This suggests that rehabilitation should not only be compensatory, but also restitutive. In other words, we should assume that children could actually relearn lost functions instead of just teaching them how to function around the loss.[31, 32]

Enriched Environments and Synapse Strengthening

Researchers now believe that neuron connections are continuously remodeled by experience, and experience is learning. For children with CVI, the learning should always follow the child's lead, be repetitive, consistent, not tiring, and positively reinforced by a parent's voice, touch, or whatever connection that can be established with the child.

One example of neuroplasticity that most parents observe is how a baby's brain changes and adapts in the first years of life. A baby's first experiences are completely sensory and feeling-oriented, and a parent understands that tenderness, touching, singing, moving, swinging are important parts of the early adaptation of a child to his environment. As the motor skills become coordinated, and speech centers develop, more neural connections, called synapses, are made. All of our knowledge and experiences are encoded into patterns of synapse strength. The more experience you have, or the more repetitive the learning behavior, as in a toddler babbling "mama" and "daddy," the more synapse strength builds.

Those synapses which are not being strengthened are pruned by the brain, and the brain keeps the synapses that are strengthened by practice, experience, and learning. This means that even if the brain has been injured in some way, new neurons can be developed and some functions can come back through consistent, repetition-type training. With intervention, the brain is flexible enough to re-learn certain things.

In extreme cases, the brain activity associated with a given function can move to a different location. In other words, if your brain gets injured in some way, the functions that the injured section of the brain used to do can actually be taken over by another area of the brain!

As Dr. Roman-Lantzy states, "The other piece that I find fascinating is that it turns out that vision can be processed all over the brain. Even when the occipital lobe is really wiped out, you can still develop vision, which is fascinating. One of the studies I am involved in with a neuro-radiologist in Pittsburgh is one in which we are actually using MRI technology to look at how kids' brains look relative to scores on the tests that I wrote, to see where this vision goes in these kids who are developing vision even when their families have been told there is no chance they could ever have this vision. Their occipital area is so damaged that they're not going to get it. Well, we do not find that to be the case. So where does vision go?"

"The brain compensates for damage by reorganizing and forming new connections between intact neurons. But, in order to reconnect, the neurons need to be stimulated through activity. Again, this is why it's so important to get a diagnosis and start intervention as early as possible."[33]

Brain Trauma and Neuroplasticity—Intervention Can Help!

"While some parts of the brain have more plastic potential because there are more neurons and connections to be altered, even non-cortical areas display plasticity."[34] The key in understanding the plasticity concept in relation to children with CVI is that training is experience specific. The more repetitive the training and the quality of your connection with your child while enjoying your time together, the more the brain will be able to adapt. Imagine a teen engrossed in playing video games every day. The more the teen enjoys the task, the more the neurons of that brain area fire and strengthen the brain structure. The same principle applies to working with our children.

With CVI, there is no question that intervention does help. As Dr. Roman-Lantzy phrased it, "For children with CVI, it is important to determine where they are on the continuum of possible impact of CVI, to identify in this way what they are able to look at or are interested in looking at, and to give them as many opportunities to look as possible by integrating motivating activities and materials into their daily lives. The goal is to facilitate looking."[35]

What this means is that with consistent intervention, a child with CVI can be taught how to translate the images that are coming into the eye into images that can be interpreted by the brain. This is all due to neuroplasticity, a concept that has done much to help our understanding and give us hope!

Dr. Roman-Lantzy shares more on the concept of neuroplasticity and age: "When I first started studying CVI and having a real interest in it, everything I read said that visual plasticity lasts for about three to seven years. By age seven, then your vision peaks and as the natural pruning of the brain implied, all of the certain pathways were formed. Even in my book, I probably say something about birth to three being optimal learning periods. No doubt that birth to three is like magic. Birth to one is really magic because of this incredible plasticity."

There is no question that early intervention is ideal. However, Dr. Roman-Lantzy emphasizes that it is never too late to intervene. Recently, her work and that of others in the field has shown, "that plasticity for vision goes on for more years than we thought, that it may even go on into adulthood. This knowledge gave me the green flag; we professionals are not going to say there is a ceiling on when this child can improve."

One study that she and her husband conducted showed that improvement in vision is more a factor of what kind of interventions a child receives than how old the child is. If your child is older or, for some reason, you were unable to intervene early on, we want you to know that there is still so much you can do!

Dr. Roman-Lantzy further emphasizes how crucial intervention is when she discusses the work of Hubel and Wiesel, "that showed us that vision really develops based on the kinds of inputs available. This intrigued me, and it was really obvious to me that children with CVI were not benefitting from the non-adapted visual world. So this child with CVI has a normal eye exam or essentially a normal eye exam. If they had detached retinas, nobody would ever diagnose CVI. These are kids whose visual problem is primarily in their brain. When one sees the child has a near-normal eye exam, one must assume that, as the child's looking out into the world, they're seeing what you see. They see all that information, but it looks like a giant hidden pictures image. It looks like nonsense. It looks like the world from their plane window at 30,000 feet. It looks like information that is so meaningless that every single element that they are viewing is perceived as novel. It does not make any sense. They do not have a springboard of knowledge from which to build in terms of their vision."

She goes on to explain, "The principle that I follow is one in which we are going to presort the environment for the child. We are going to start with the things that are very familiar to the child. We are going to present them in certain ways. We are going to add movement or light, certain colors, just to help the child remember what they saw. After which, we build from there so that the child develops a bigger repertoire of skills, and over time as they grow and increase their functional vision, they can actually handle more complexity, and they can recognize that object at greater distances, and they can recognize that object even when it is not exactly the same."

"Children build visual schemes. They are really developing visual schema, and it turns out that this plasticity process, it just does not seem to be linked in a real specific way to age. Anecdotally, from the data we have collected, the younger children seem to improve faster than the older children."

"But I really also think that if you are ten years old and nobody has ever worked specifically around your CVI needs, and you have developed other ways of interacting with the world through touch and sound, it is pretty hard to change. You get resistant to someone saying, now, instead of that, we want you to do this. There is a human resistance that also interferes at that point. We do not know if that is purely plasticity, or whether it is plasticity and previous learning that has the child kind of stumped about why you want them now to try another method."

According to Dr. Roman-Lantzy, the first step in her work is to identify where a child is on the CVI Range, which she discusses in depth in her book, *Cortical Visual Impairment: An Approach to Assessment and Intervention*. She continues, "The assessment that I wrote is designed specifically for kids with CVI to figure out what level of CVI they have. Then build an intervention program, a support program, and adaptations to environments and materials that are based on solely that score. This score is like the child's corrective lenses. You do not want their lenses to be too weak or too strong. You want to bring it to the place where they see best. Then those activities, those interventions must be paired with meaningful, functional, real activities throughout the day because frequency seems to be very important. So that's the bottom line."[36]

For this reason, it is important to find professionals to work with your child who understand CVI. Getting a proper assessment is vital to creating appropriate intervention strategies that will meet your child where she is. Tapping into neuroplasticity in terms of CVI is not about presenting your child with visual information that is too complex, but about adapting their world so that they can use the visual skills they already have. As opportunities to use vision increase, those skills will also increase and the characteristics of CVI will begin to resolve. Even if you don't have an official diagnosis from a doctor, it is important to learn as much as you can about CVI and about your child's specific abilities so that you can begin to tap into the amazing plasticity of the brain!

9

What to Do: Strategies for Helping Your Child Learn to See

Believe. No pessimist ever discovered the secrets of the stars,
or sailed to an uncharted land, or opened a new heaven
to the human spirit.

Helen Keller

Strategies Must Be Functional

You have read the stories of the medical evaluations that some families of children with CVI have experienced. Such assessments can tell parents which area of the brain is injured, levels of visual acuity, and help a doctor diagnose CVI and accompanying conditions. It is important to have your child examined by a medical professional, but it is also important to remember that many medical professionals don't yet know much about CVI. If you suspect your child has CVI, you can begin intervention even without an official diagnosis from a doctor. Intervention therapists, such as teachers of the visually impaired (TVIs), and educators who are knowledgeable about CVI can determine a child's functional vision and develop educational strategies for children with CVI.

You may find professionals like therapists and teachers who are not completely familiar with the differences in children who have CVI and children with other visual impairments. We have covered the topic previously and summarize it here for your review. Remember that your child may have some or all of these features:

Children with CVI	Children with Ocular Impairment
Normal eye exam (unless some kind of ocular impairment is co-occurring)	Abnormal eye exam
Inconsistent visual functioning	Consistent visual functions
Short visual attention span	Consistent attention span
Coordinated eye movements	Observable lack of coordinated eye movements
Compulsive light-gazing	No compulsive gazing at light
No eye-pressing	Eye-pressing
Has color perception	May not have color perception,

To determine the functional vision of children with CVI, Dr. Christine Roman-Lantzy developed an assessment and intervention tool known as *The CVI Range* to measure skills and progress in the functional vision of children with CVI. Through techniques of observation and interview, usually of the parents, and/or a teacher or therapist, the tool evaluates the level of visual function and the effects of CVI on visual function. The common characteristics of CVI are listed here as a review, and you can refer to chapter 6 for more detail. The characteristics of a child with CVI are: color preferences, movement preference, field preferences, difficulty with visual complexity, visual latency, light-gazing and nonpurposeful gazing behaviors, trouble with distance viewing, absent or atypical visual reflexes, difficulties with visual novelty and coordination of guided reach.

As we mentioned in chapter 6, Dr. Roman-Lantzy divides CVI into three phases. The majority of children will start in Phase I and are likely to have most of the CVI characteristics. The CVI characteristics start to be corrected or resolved as the child moves through Phase II, and by the time they have reached the end of Phase III, the child can display near-normal vision. These skill progressions do not happen overnight, but can take several years. Intervention strategies produce progressive results in functional vision as reported by the following Pediatric View Study: *"Data collected in the Pediatric View study suggest that functional vision in individuals who have CVI can be measured and that improvements in functional vision are not simply associated with a child getting older or with the child's neurological history."*[37]

Intervention Strategies

For a child with CVI, it is crucial to follow the child's lead. Find objects and activities of visual interest and cognitive interest. If materials are not motivating the child, then use other materials. Once you know where your child falls on the CVI range, you will be better able to create opportunities for him to use his vision. Note your child's responses to each adaptation you make to the environment. Does the child's vision improve when you reduce distractions such as sound or visual clutter? Does he pay attention to red objects but not to blue? Does he need movement or light in order to notice an object? All of these observations will help you learn the best ways to facilitate vision in your child. We will review ways to work with the various characteristics below.

As we have mentioned before, opportunities to use vision should be incorporated into your child's everyday life. For example, if red is your child's preferred color, you might use a red bowl or plate for each meal. Adding a red ribbon to a bottle for younger children works well. You could also place a red object on or near the diaper changing table, car seat or wheelchair. You can ask your child's other therapists to wear red clothes when working with him. Our physical therapist, for example, often wears long red gloves when working with Little Bear so he can more easily see her hands and arms. The key is to place opportunities for the child to see throughout their daily routine. It becomes easier and easier for kids with CVI to see these objects as the child becomes familiar with them. It can also be helpful to keep one familiar object, like a yellow Big Bird doll, with your child throughout the day. This allows the child to learn to recognize the object in different environments. Furthermore, children with CVI may tire easily when engaged in visual tasks, which is another reason to keep vision sessions short and frequent throughout the day.

Because latency is a common characteristic of CVI, children often need a lot of time to respond visually. When presenting an object, remember that you may need to wait several minutes before seeing a response. This is especially true of unfamiliar objects. When we first started working with Little Bear he would look at objects for only a second at a time before looking away. What was important was that he would return to the object repeatedly.

It is also important to remember that it will be much easier for your child to see if she is properly positioned. This means giving a child as much support as possible. For example, a child who has to work to hold up her head will be less able to focus on using her vision. Little Bear seems to use his vision best when lying on his back or being held in a sitting position.

Look for visual field preferences and place objects according to the child's needs. There is no rule as to whether central vision or peripheral vision is better. Try placing the object in different areas to learn where your child sees best.

Rather than just placing an object in a child's hands, guide the child's hand to the object or tease the child to reach by touching the object to his fingers for exploration. If your child is not yet reaching for toys, try to incorporate items that she can feel and see simultaneously.

Before Little Bear learned to reach for toys, we would use items like a yellow slinky, which we could hold high enough that it was in his preferred field of vision, but dangled low enough that he could still feel it easily. Long chains of beads, large stuffed animals and plastic leis are also useful for this purpose.

For children who are sensitive to light, place them with their back to the light, or use indirect lighting with little glare or reflection. If sensitive to bright sunlight, protective shades on the eyes or in a car window when travelling are helpful.

Remember that light can also be used to get a child's attention. In a dark room or at night, try shining a flashlight on the object you wish the child to see. Brightly colored glow sticks are great for kids who like light and they are often small enough and lightweight enough that even kids with limited muscle strength can easily hold on to them. As we discussed in chapter 6, light boxes and iPads are also great ways to incorporate light into visual activities.

Establish an uncluttered physical space for visual learning. The space can include a dark background of some kind, familiar objects of the preferred color, lights, and even pictures and numbers for older children. Remember not to overload the space with items, however. Keep it simple. Watch for your child's visual preferences when placing a picture or objects.

In order to maximize your child's ability to use vision throughout the day, it is important to provide several spaces, based on routine, that are free of distractions and visual clutter. Learning to see can be very taxing and difficult for a child with CVI. If the environment is too visually complex or contains competing sensory input it can be difficult for the child to focus on vision. You can reduce visual clutter by providing an all-black background against which shiny, bright objects with highly saturated colors are placed. Reduce other stimulation if you find that your child is too sensitive to noise, bright lighting, or is easily fatigued by people and talking in the environment.

Pair cues in a consistent way to your intervention, to increase familiarity and routine. One verbal example is Geetha saying to her son during bath time each day, "I am going to wipe your eyes now, one, two, three, four." He closes his eyes on the cue of four. Coordinate looking and listening activities carefully when using intervention with your child. Sound can be distracting if you are using visual stimulus and you want the child to concentrate on looking. Use your child's listening skills as an adjunct to visual activities. Whatever lesson or activity you begin, use visual stimulus first before talking. Make sound a powerful reinforcement to looking. For example, after Lukas looks at his Elmo doll, we may sing or talk to reward him and reinforce his looking.

Pairing a touch on the shoulder, caress of the arm or tactile tenderness during presentation of a book with large pictures or colorful objects can also be a pleasurable way to build the desire to repeat the bonding and learning. Particularly in the beginning, use real objects rather than pictures of objects as two-dimensional items are often more difficult for kids with CVI to see.

Use touch cues for sound-sensitive children to train your child to understand the daily routines. For example, two taps on the under-arms could indicate being picked up. Paired with speech, the cues help children be less anxious as they mature and enter new situations.

Since a child's brain is wired for movement, some moms have shared that their child with CVI enjoys watching golf on television. Another dad shakes each toy or object first, then holds it still, and then re-shakes the object for visual attention and focus. While we prefer to take Little Bear to the aquarium to watch the movement of the fish and water up close, we did find suggestions for television viewing for children with CVI on the Scottish Sensory Center web site (www.ssc.education.ed.ac.uk). The suggestions included using a large screen TV to help compensate for poor acuity and visual crowding and using flat screen TVs, which have better contrast. Also, "allow the child to sit up close to the TV so that surrounding visual clutter is minimized."[38] Choosing programs that are visually simpler and contain bright colors can also be helpful. Try different shows to see what your child enjoys.

Orientation Strategies

No matter how old your child with CVI may be, you can be aware of how to guide your child through or adapt your home environment for easier movement. Also, your child may have mobility or orientation training as part of her intervention plan or educational plan, but you will still need to implement many strategies at home as part of your child's intervention team. Our suggestions can get you started, and are by no means all-inclusive.

Some parents have reported their children's difficulties with stairs and adaptation options include tactile guidance or color guidance. Tactile guidance can include several enhancements to guide the movement up or down. For example, you can add texture on the handrails, a strip of textured paint at hand height to guide the child up the stairs, or textured stair treads or mats on each step, which guide the way up or down the stairs.

Color enhancements can also be effective in several ways. A stripe of bright paint, a color your child recognizes, can also guide the way up or down the steps. Brightly colored stair treads or a flat surfaced bright circle, square or even shoe print painted in the center can offer visual clues.

Another strategy to consider is training the child to go up and down the stairs by facing straight ahead and letting his sense of his own body guide the motions of his feet. It takes practice, almost like a drill, to learn the way to lift the feet and use the arms, if possible, for light touch along the wall; but once learned, the child will not forget. Spot-lighting each step also helps with visual training and feet placement.

Coming down the steps is typically more difficult for children than going up. Depending on the child's ability to physically shift, you may want to start your child's journey in steps training by having her sit on the upper step and slide down one step at a time. Again, using the whole body will more physically support the sense of her body in space and movement. This method provides confidence rather than fear of the unknown.

Most literature that we have read includes suggestions for removing patterned carpets, colored tiles and uneven floor surfaces of brick or wood. Laminated flooring, smooth and flat surfaces, and no inclines work best for children with CVI.

For children whose impairment leaves them bumping into walls, you can adapt the furniture or doors by following a few simple guidelines. A fun idea for children is to use a set of footprints, which guides the child from one room to another and creates a trail through the center of rooms and doorways or along the side of a room—wherever you want them to walk. If texture helps your child's footing, then use textured paper, paint or even colorful bathtub stickers of solid bright colors that contrast with the floor.

The use of florescent paint or paint in your child's preferred color can help in several ways: to highlight the edges of the stairs on both sides; to highlight the handrail on the stairs; to color the baseboards in a well-used room to provide a visual floor plan; to paint doors or door frames as a boundary definition or visual clue to slow down, making movement easier.

Other environmental suggestions fall into the common sense realm depending upon your family's lifestyle. Minimizing furniture and making sure there are high color contrasts between furniture and the floor or carpet can be helpful. Eliminate sharp corners, glass, stone furniture, metal railings, knick-knacks that break easily or any element that can hurt a child if he falls into or against it. If your child with CVI bumps into doors or doorframes, two options are to paint the doors a bright color, or to remove them altogether, depending upon the flow of traffic. Additionally, nothing works as well as guided training to assist in the development of familiar pathways.

The parents' stories in this book reflect how they have adapted the environment to help their children with CVI. They incorporate therapeutic tasks into their daily routines. Adapting life for a child with CVI requires creativity and is even more important now that neuroplasticity research is showing the regeneration of neural pathways is possible. For you, it means all that you are doing is an absolutely positive contribution to your child's brain education and orientation to life.

10
The Williams' Advocating

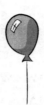

There should be some special award for these parents who manage to deepen their love with this (CVI) challenge.[39]

Leah Williams' Story

Krista Williams is a staunch advocate for her six-year-old daughter Leah, who has acquired cortical visual impairment. Krista delivered Leah through normal full-term birth. Brandon and Krista brought their baby girl home and she thrived for the first five and a half months. One afternoon, Leah's great-great grandma was speaking to her while she was propped up in a corner of the loveseat, and Leah's eyes kept rolling up to the right.

Krista worked in a pediatrician's office. At work the next day, during lunchtime, she spoke to the doctor. After Krista explained Leah's eye's rolling, the doctor agreed to check on the condition.

The next morning, Krista took Leah into the doctor's office before hours. The pediatrician found Leah was not tracking with one eye. Another pediatrician was asked to look at Leah and he added, "No, she's not tracking with that eye at all." The pediatrician called and spoke to the ophthalmologist at the local children's hospital, two hours away, and set an immediate appointment for Krista and Leah. After an examination, the ophthalmologist believed Leah had a little delayed maturation of her vision that would get better over time since Leah was tracking with one eye.

The eye rolling and lack of visual tracking with one eye was the very first thing that was noticed. Yet, Krista was not comfortable with the diagnosis. Brandon thought she was worrying herself over nothing and said, "See, I told you there is nothing wrong."

Krista again expressed concern to the pediatrician, "There's something not right. I do not know what it is, but something is not right. I know you are not supposed to compare kids, but she is just different from her brothers."

"Well, do you think maybe she is autistic or something?"

"I do not know. Call it mother's intuition, but I cannot let it go."

"Well, let me refer you to a neurodevelopmental pediatrician." They set an appointment for two weeks later.

In the meantime, Krista took Leah back into the pediatrician for her six-month check-up, and by then, Leah had completely stopped tracking with both eyes. With trepidation, the pediatrician said, "Krista, I think she is blind. Leah has no threat reflex, no blink reflex, nothing. There is nothing there visually anymore."

Krista shares, "Deep down, I knew something was not right. But I am a get-it-done person. The next day at work, I was on the internet, and I put in all of Leah's symptoms: no visual tracking, blind, eye rolling. A CVI checklist came up. I looked through it, and I knew this was totally Leah. The office staff thought somebody died because I just cried and cried. I printed it out the checklist and I took it to the pediatrician."

"I was scared, but also relieved. I thought my daughter was blind. The checklist described her vision as looking through a piece of Swiss cheese. Perhaps she really could see some things. I was also happy because we thought she was completely blind, and maybe she could see. Though we did not fight, my husband and I were on different pages."

"I kept searching. The checklist of CVI symptoms answered the question deep in my gut about what Leah's symptoms meant. Our next step was to see Dr. Marla Moon, a low vision specialist in State College, Pennsylvania. I remember the doctor watching Leah. She had some kind of a thing that lit up and she was trying to get Leah to track. She kept doing it over and over and over again. I did not tell her anything about cortical visual impairment, and my pediatrician did not either, as she just wanted a low vision evaluation. After a time of watching Dr. Moon, I finally spoke up, 'I think I know what is wrong with her.'

'You do?' She spun around on her stool, looked at me and said, 'What is that?'

'I think she has cortical visual impairment.'

She just looked at me and said, 'That is exactly what she has.'"

"So, Leah finally received her official diagnosis at six-and-a-half months of age. Dr. Marla's recommendations included Early Intervention, to get a teacher of the visually impaired to start working with Leah, and to get a light box with Level I materials from the American Printing House for the Blind."

Like most parents who first learn of a diagnosis, Krista followed the suggestions provided by her physician, knowing nothing about what a light box was or anything about organizations for the blind. Krista's journey to being her daughter's advocate, and an advocate for all other families she would meet in the coming years, started when she walked out of Dr. Moon's office.

Krista continues, "What was a light box? Our caseworker told us that getting a light box was like platinum, and it was really hard to do. This was the beginning of me learning to advocate, because never in a million years would I have imagined that you have to advocate as much as you do for your child."

"You have to network, and you have to know how to network. If you do not receive an answer or reply, you have to go to the next person up, even if you have to go to a supervisor's supervisor. You keep accurate notes and documentation of when you call, whom you call, whom you talk to and what they said. You just have to fight for what your child needs."

"Once Leah got her diagnosis, she was able to get on our state insurance, Medicaid. Her insurance was Medicaid and because Blindness and Visual Services is also a state-run program, I contacted our local state representative and talked to a lady at his office and simply asked, 'Is there any way you can help us?'"

"Dr. Moon really expressed that the biggest step for Leah visually was to stimulate her vision. I wanted to get as much vision or processing ability as we could for Leah. They asked me to write a letter. Once I wrote them a letter, within three days we received two light boxes; one came from the insurance company and one came from Blindness and Visual Services."

"Two weeks after we saw Dr. Moon, our next appointment was with the neurodevelopmental pediatrician. By then, Leah had regressed completely. She did not move. She only stared at lights, making no eye contact. It was almost like socially she was not there anymore because she did not interact with anyone."

"Leah's MRI showed some demyelination of the brain, which is normal for a child of that age. After many other tests, he referred us to a neurologist. Before that appointment, I was sitting on the couch at home holding Leah and she started rhythmically throwing her arms and legs every eight seconds. I counted it. So I will never forget, every eight seconds she would do it over and over and over again."

"I knew she was having a seizure, and I called my aunt because we did not have internet at the time. I said, 'Hey, I need you to look this up for me.' My aunt eventually found something called West Syndrome, a term used in European communities. In the Unites States, it is infantile spasms."

"The next morning, I heard the doctor come in, and I went back to her office and said, 'Hey, I think I know what is going on with Leah.'

'You do? What's that?'

'I think she has West Syndrome.'

'West Syndrome? That's infantile spasms. What do you mean? You think she has infantile spasms?'

'Yeah, I think she had a seizure last night.' I described the seizure to her.

'Oh, my gosh. That is it exactly. I bet you that is what it is.' She got right on the phone to the neurologist that Leah was scheduled with and the neurologist explained that kids with infantile spasms show a specific pattern on their EEG called hypsarrhythmia. Only kids with infantile spasms have hypsarrhythmia, and sometimes it takes a while for that to actually show on EEG so waiting two weeks until her appointment would be okay."

"In those two weeks, Leah was having seizures eighteen hours out of the day. They did the EEG and they did a visual evoked potential (VEP), because of the cortical visual impairment. When the technician left the room, I already knew something was wrong. Next they tested Leah's hearing with an ABR test, and we went to lunch and returned."

"When the neurologist came in and sat down, she said, 'your suspicions were right, it is definitely infantile spasms. I need you to go home, make arrangements, pack clothes, and I need you to come back tomorrow. We are going to admit her and start her on a steroid shot called ATCH, which is one of three treatments for infantile spasms.' The treatment worked, and I really did not think it was going to work since the spasms were so bad."

Leah was seizure-free for four years, and then she started having complex partial seizures on the right side of her body at age five. Like Leah, most kids with infantile spasms end up having another form of seizure disorder at some point in time.

"Leah actually had seizures up until twelve weeks ago. When she started having seizures, her eating got worse. She did not eat or drink well. We tried Pediasure, Pediasure 1.5, which has one-and-a-half times the calories as regular Pediasure, and we could not get her to gain weight. As things got worse, last spring she contracted pneumonia, and it seemed like everything was downhill from there. We talked about a feeding tube because when she stopped eating and drinking, and barely ate and drank for four and five days at a time, her seizures would disappear. I wondered at the correlation between food and seizures, which I mentioned to the neurologist. Leah would either stop having them or they lessened when she did not eat. So her neurologist mentioned starting her on the Ketogenic Diet,[4040] "Ketogenic Diet." *Epilepsy Foundation*, . a diet high in fat and low in carbs. The Ketogenic Diet makes your brain burn fat instead of sugar and glucose, and it worked. She has not had a seizure since November 8, 2011."

"On the Ketogenic Diet, we weigh everything on a gram scale. Leah's meals are very tiny. When she was on the feeding tube over the summer, we noticed that when we were putting Pediasure through her feeding tube, her seizures were getting worse. Her body mass index was down below 5 percent, to the point of malnourishment. So we had to get her nourishment up first before we could even do the diet, which has been a challenge with some GI Issues. The past month has been pretty good for her."

Leah's Educational Program—Managing the Shuffle

Krista explains how the family's adapted. "Through the Early Intervention Program, Leah was receiving five hours of therapy weekly. When I worked, and they were here, I missed all their instructions, which Brandon and I were to supplement. I had a learning curve after I quit my job. I pretty much took Leah on, and Brandon helped with Leah, but he also inherited the boys and their sports activities."

"Early Intervention worked with Leah consistently until she turned three, and then she went to preschool at the local preschool, where she first started out in an integrated classroom. In this school district, integrated classrooms consist of five children with disabilities and five children without disabilities learning together. We discovered that the classroom was too busy for Leah. She likes noise, but for her to be able to focus visually, there was way too much going on for her. There was an opening in a communication disorders' classroom where the majority of the kids were autistic and pretty non-verbal. The environment was quieter for Leah, more structured. This was the best placement for her for what was available in our pretty rural area."

"New therapists came into the home about six months before Leah started preschool. They started questioning why we did activities a certain way. For example, rather than doing the straight therapies, my routines and play with Leah developed around what she needed. Like feeding her, we would sit her in her highchair and spread her Cheerios out. She would have to use her eyes and look to pick up Cheerios, instead of feeling for a clump of Cheerios she could pick up without looking." Krista wasn't aware of how she was adapting her family's routines to meet Leah's needs until the therapists pointed it out. They showed her more ways to help Leah.

"We also learned a lot of accommodation. Many stores have special-needs toys out there, but are very expensive. However, we took regular toys and altered them. For example, we changed our swing set. The ladder looks like rocks that you have to climb up. There are flat pieces where your feet are supposed to go. Leah would not even look to see where her feet went, but she was persistent and kept trying, unsuccessfully."

"We had to bring Leah's attention to be able to see those flat pieces and learn to go up and down on her own. I bought gold Mylar sticky paper, cut them to the size of a curved area on the flat-looking steps. After three days, she was able to go up the ladder by herself because she could visually look and know where to put her feet and her hands to be able to climb. We adapted the environment for her. She learned to do it by herself, and eventually the sticky paper blew away."

Receiving Help for the CVI Diagnosis

Dr. Moon mentioned Dr. Roman to Krista on the day she diagnosed Leah, but Krista did not remember with all the overwhelming activity. She saw other parents on the internet mention Dr. Roman, and discovered she was only three hours away.

Krista shares her advocacy, "The reason I was looking for Dr. Roman before Leah was almost two was because her ophthalmologist was still calling her condition delayed visual maturation. By then, Leah's vision had improved a lot. After her seizures were controlled, her CVI improved and went from Phase I to the beginning of Phase II just by seizure control and intervention. Just before Christmas, when she was diagnosed, she started tracking with one eye. Shortly after Christmas, she started tracking with her other eye."

"I was just frustrated with the ophthalmologist. He told me CVI does not get better. He insisted that Leah could not have CVI because it does not get better. I knew better. I had researched it enough. All I needed was for him to check her eyes, to make sure the structure was okay, but I still had conflicting diagnoses and I wanted to know. I thought she had CVI. Dr. Moon thought she had it. The ophthalmologist at the children's hospital was saying no, it does not get better. I wanted Dr. Roman to give me a straight answer. Finally, we saw Dr. Roman in March 2007, when Leah was just shy of two."

"We met with Dr. Roman and her husband. She told us, and I never thought of it this way, that Leah has acquired cortical visual impairment, because her vision was normal before, but she acquired it because of the infantile spasms. Several weeks later, I attended Dr. Roman's three-day training with Leah's vision teacher. I learned all about CVI, and a light bulb went on for me. I could not figure out why Leah always tripped over our white cat, yet she could see a Cheerio on the floor. Dr. Roman told a story about observing a little child at his school. The boy was running around and was tripping over people. Then she mentioned that pretty much every child she has ever met with CVI has a lower field issue. I looked at her vision teacher and we both knew finally that Leah was tripping over the cat because of the lower field problem. That also explained why Leah had issues going up and down stairs."

"So we followed up with Dr. Roman for years. Once Leah transitioned to preschool, I thought to have our intermediate unit (IU) do training on CVI because these specialists knew nothing about it. They fought me on it, but I advocated, went to the next supervisor, and they did training on cortical visual impairment at our local intermediate unit. To this day, it was the biggest training they have ever had."

"During Leah's next school year, she was meeting her Individualized Education Program (IEP) goals at a very slow rate, and no one knew how to help her. The IU brought Dr. Roman up, and she observed Leah in the classroom and then in her therapies, and gave the teachers and therapists recommendations and ideas for adaptations. Then she did another training the next day, again at the IU for a larger group of therapists."

"Since then, Leah has made the most developmental progress ever by her teachers adapting the environment to her needs . . . like getting rid of complexity, using a simple background for presentation. They created a vision corner with black backgrounds to work with her. They have a closet to work in with kids, and Leah focused better without the visual distractions. Also Leah actually works better in briefer periods, and under this condition, therapists have a better response from Leah. She stays focused and does not get as aggravated. Adapting the environment has really made a difference!"

You have read the stories of different families seeking the help they need for their children with CVI. In the next chapter, you will learn more about early intervention and school programs and how they can assist your child.

11

Moving Through Education Systems

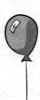

It is only by careful assessment and continued observation of the visual behaviour of such children that we can gain a deeper understanding of how they see. This knowledge can in turn be used to structure communication, information and the environment to enhance the child's social skills, learning and mobility by ensuring that each element is designed to fall within the perceptual limitations of each child.[41]

The Parent Is the First Teacher

You know your child well, and from the first time, or even before, you received the CVI diagnosis, you spent time and became intimate with your child's behaviors and moods. You are the most accurate reporter that professionals can rely on for feedback and suggestions to help them learn about your child and her needs. Here are some suggestions to help you in your role as expert:

• From day one keep documented notes on medical conditions, prescriptions, doctors' visits and diagnoses.

- Keep a diary of your child's obvious behaviors, such as light-gazing, but also about the subtle behaviors such as a glance, a response, a preference, a favorite position, toy, color or food.

- Include in your notes any of your child's sensitivities to sound, movement, or other distractions in the environment, clothing, touch, etc.

- Note what you observe about your child's fatigue level when you go through your routines each day.

It is crucial that all team members understand that the complex physical and neuropsychological aspect of seeing profoundly affects the child's mobility, emotionality, and ability to communicate. Thus, all educational goals should aim toward guiding the child with CVI to functionality in vision tasks, movement, communication, and living skills.

In summary, a parent may find her or himself continually educating a child's team about their child with CVI, and asking for agreement that they work from the premise of plasticity in continually observing and assessing new skills and celebrating accomplishments. It may seem daunting at first, but over time you will adapt to your role as advocate and teacher.

Team Members You May Meet Along the Way

Neonatal Intensive Care Units (NICU) offer medical support for premature or sick babies. Parents may be in crisis mode and need to understand what their baby is experiencing and what their medical options are. Over time, and with stabilization of your child's condition, you will learn what to expect and how to respond to your baby.

We bonded with Lukas in the NICU despite the many machines and tubes he was connected to. In the beginning, we felt more like dispensers of medicines and keepers of schedules than parents. The nurses and caseworkers provided updates about our son, but some also offered support, understanding and ideas about how to help him.

Unlike our experience, the Champine family knew Carson would be born with some difficulties, and the caseworker from the hospice program made home visits to provide support for Kevin, Alicia and Carson. When Carson grew and thrived, they moved ahead with therapeutic care for him. The hospice caseworker located a vision therapist knowledgeable about CVI, and the Champine family incorporated her suggestions about CVI into their daily routines.

If life with your child starts out in the NICU, you will find that a caseworker or an assigned nurse can help stabilize your family through the transition from NICU to home. Social workers, counselors or therapists can also help you to cope through this incredibly difficult time. At this point, the assistance will likely be more medical than educational in offering support when you transition home.

If you live in the US, in most cases, you will be referred to an Early Intervention Program. Ask for this referral as soon as you can as it may take some time before therapy actually begins. Learn as much as you can so that you can begin to help your child as early as possible.

Agreements among Team Members

Whether your child with CVI is an infant, a preschooler or older, there will be a continued team of professionals who work with you in helping your child acquire and maintain skill levels. Insure that your team agrees they are working with the mechanism of plasticity in order to educate the brain. If you find therapists who do not believe this, or they are of the old school that brain damage is irreparable, or their work with your child seems perfunctory and without enthusiasm, find another therapist.

We cannot urge you strongly enough to find a medical doctor who hears you and acknowledges your concerns, or a case worker who is your proponent in the maze of insurance, medical, and educational systems, or knowledgeable and well-trained therapists or teachers who know your child's needs and how to provide for those needs.

Your role as parent also means you are the automatic advocate for your child. You may have to, for example, act as Krista Williams did and bring the training directly to your child's teachers and therapists if they do not know how to work with your child. Like us, you may not actually have an official CVI diagnosis and you may have to be the one to convince your child's doctors that he does, in fact, have CVI.

By using the concept of plasticity as a team guideline for educational support, therapists and teachers will understand what a child with CVI needs. CVI intervention should include:

• Consistent and repetitive visual function and/or visual motor skill-building

• Planning to meet the child's specific needs within specific routines

• A high frequency of presentations

• A design for comfort, familiarity, and connected interactions throughout the child's day

This team approach is actually easier to implement than it first appears. Therapists will have scheduled times with your child, but you, as a parent, can take their ideas and suggestions and incorporate them into your child's day; for example, doing stretching on the floor mat or changing table as Alicia Champine did with Carson. Visual skill-building should be functional and tied in with life development skills such as helping your child to see their food, play with toys, know where they are in space and learn to move around your home, or negotiate stairs.

As Dr. Roman-Lantzy reminded us previously, long educational sessions are not necessarily better than those of short duration. The key for the child is that short sessions are frequent and familiar. The fun for the child is in a positive connection that helps him want to learn. Parents can remind professionals to not have judgment about why a child is not learning a skill, or naming a child's behaviors as negative because the child is not responding to a lesson, material, or person. Patience and persistence are keys.

A professional who has no training in CVI may not understand the reasons that a child with CVI may not perform a task or show interest in skill development. The child may be fatigued, the environment may be too distracting, or there may be neurological or other health conditions getting in the way. Many parents of a child with CVI have spent long hours in observation and play to notice when and how their child responds to them. You are the expert on your child and your input is invaluable to your child's team.

Next we will discuss the Early Intervention and Special Education Programs that are available in the United States in more detail. While this information can get you started, it is by no means exhaustive. Be sure to familiarize yourself with all the resources available in your community.

Individuals with Disabilities Education Act (IDEA)

(This section is relevant to programs in the United States and territories.)

First, we will provide a brief history of the Early Intervention Programs, as not everyone is aware of services that may be available through their state or local educational agencies. We will acquaint you with terms to know as your child enters the educational system or the special education programs available to you.

In the United States, the special education law is titled *The Individuals with Disabilities Education Act* (IDEA) and is implemented in all states and U. S. territories on local levels. The purpose of IDEA is to provide guidelines for the education of children with disabilities. State education agencies, regional education agencies and your local special education program in your school district implement these guidelines through programs and services for children with disabilities. In addition, there may be local programs, coordinated with hospitals, or private therapists who participate in the planning for a child's educational or therapeutic services unique to his needs.

Each child receiving special education services is required to have an Individualized Education Program (IEP), in which all service providers, as well as parents, agree upon common assessments, educational goals, planned intervention or educational activities, classroom placement, and how and when a child's progress will be evaluated.

Part C of IDEA provides guidelines for the Early Intervention Programs for children, from birth to age three, with significant developmental delay or disability. However, instead of an individualized education plan, a family that qualifies and receives services from Early Intervention will have an Individual Family Service Plan (IFSP), which recognizes the parents as the child's first teacher.

We found the web site of the National Dissemination Center for Children with Disabilities (www.nichcy.org) most helpful if you wish to find the criteria for eligibility of visual impairment. The following page (www.nichcy.org/disability/specific/visualimpairment) offers information about state and national organizations and a sample Individual Family Service Plan. It can also help you understand what is expected of you as the parent, and learn about early intervention strategies and outcomes.

Intervention through the Early Intervention Programs first requires a case worker or case manager who coordinates the intervention serv-ices and is your go-to person for all questions, material requests, and counseling support. Services can also include:

• Family training, counseling, and home visits

• Teachers of the visually impaired (TVI)

• Speech-language pathology services (sometimes referred to as speech therapy)

• Audiology services (hearing impairment services)

• Occupational therapy

• Physical therapy

• Psychological services; medical services (only for diagnostic or evaluation purposes)

• Health services needed to enable your child to benefit from the other services

• Social work services

• Assistive technology devices and services

• Transportation

• Nutrition services

• Service coordination services.[42]

In summary, your baby, toddler or young child with CVI may be referred to and assessed by members of your local Early Intervention Program. An Individual Family Services Plan will describe results of assessments, services to be provided and the expected results of those services. Most likely, services can be provided directly to the child in your home, so that you can incorporate skill building into your family routines to insure practical application. Family education is an important part of the programs.

Here are some questions you may want to ask to insure you have the right therapists who understand your child:

- Are you knowledgeable specifically about cortical visual impairment?

- Are you knowledgeable about associated medical conditions of my child?

- Are you aware that the main problem for children with CVI is in the area of brain injury, not the eye itself?

- Do you know the importance of vision in the normal development of a child and how visual impairment impacts development?

- Do you know how to integrate sensory information for sensory enhancement into my child's therapies?

- Do you know how to adapt or structure the environment to enhance my child's learning?

- What assistive devices does my child need? How do I obtain those?

- What materials and tools are available to us through you?

- What communication technology, if any, can my child benefit from, and how do I obtain that technology?

Transitioning from Early Intervention to Special Education

School districts in the United States provide special education services for children in the age range of three to five in preschool programs. Eligibility falls under the same guidelines as Early Intervention, which provides for children with a disability or developmental delay. Your child may continue to undergo assessments to gauge her learning progress in terms of goals, and may also have further assessments in these areas:

• Physical development (fine motor skills, gross motor skills)

• Cognitive development (intellectual abilities)

• Communication development (speech and language)

• Social or emotional development (social skills, emotional control)

• Adaptive development (self-care skills)

Now that your child with CVI is going to school, the Individualized Education Program (IEP) replaces the Individual Family Services Plan (IFSP). The same types of services are available as on the Early Intervention list, but therapy services such as speech therapy or vision therapy now take place in a classroom. Your child will also have a classroom teacher, who will most likely serve as IEP team leader and coordinator of the child's educational program. The IEP team members are therapists or specialists who will integrate your child into the classroom through "specially designed instruction, which is adapting the content, methodology, or delivery of instruction."[43]

If your child needs specific accommodations or support, remember that you are an integral part of the IEP team and can request, "adapted equipment—such as a special seat or a cut-out cup for drinking; assistive technology—such as a word processor, special software, or a communication system; training for staff, student, and/or parents; peer tutors; a one-on-one aide; adapted materials—such as books on tape, large print, or highlighted notes; or collaboration/consultation among staff, parents, and/or other professionals."[44]

Be the advocate, like Krista Williams who, as a parent member of her daughter's IEP team, requested that she and her vision teacher, as well as others, be able to take the CVI training offered by Dr. Roman-Lantzy in order to make appropriate classroom accommodations for Leah. Krista also suggests that you think about what you need to know from the school as a parent. For example, a communication book between teachers and parents tells the parents which IEP goals your child worked on that day and how they progressed. Ask yourself if there is any other specific information you need a report on: visits to the school nurse, food preferences, allergies or meal intake, visits with the sighted children in the regular classroom and so on.

After Age 5

Experts say that roughly 80 percent of what a child learns in school is information that is presented visually.[45] School-aged children with visual problems or impairments of the eye itself are likely to find that these problems interfere with learning. Your child with CVI will continue to use the special education services in grade school and onward, depending on how your school district provides for accommodations of your child's needs. Your child will gain skills and move to other educational goals appropriate to his age and grade, but remember that environmental adaptation becomes increasingly important.

Does your child have fatigue issues, a continued need for low lights, quieter environments, vision learning areas, an iPad or other technology devices, mobility training, continued therapeutic services in

OT, PT or speech? Will these be best accommodated through inclusion with more typical kids, or with other students with disabilities? As Krista mentioned, her daughter Leah started in a classroom with five children with disabilities and five without disabilities. The noise level for her was less distracting in a classroom for only children with disabilities. Also, your child's social needs are a consideration as she matures. Be aware of all of your child's needs and communicate them to the rest of the team. You are your child's primary advocate.

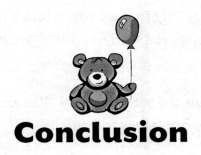

Conclusion

When it is dark enough, you can see the stars.
Ralph Waldo Emerson

We wrote this book for you. Our Little Bear and other families and children with CVI we have met along the way have inspired us. We have learned that in the midst of these challenges, there is so much hope, so much beauty and so much love. This encouraged us to reach out and share stories, ideas and resources. Truly, we are on this walk together! Although we email, talk on the phone, or like each other on Facebook, we can easily forget in our daily routines, advocacy, medical and therapy appointments, that we are not alone.

We must change the face of CVI as it is today—a new field with a handful of courageous professionals who are writing, teaching, educating and helping, though still a field that many doctors, therapists and parents know little about. As parents, we must also step up and share our hearts and support; to write, teach, and educate each other and those new parents out there facing what we have faced.

We are our children's first teachers. We do know them intimately and understand how they learn and what they need. We also believe in them and know they can do so much, much more!

We hope this book has informed you and inspired you in some way to pay your heart forward to the next parent who has questions and who needs understanding. Together we will create a network of informed parents who can change the field of cortical visual impairment as it is today.

Remember, we all walk the same journey. We can find hope and inspiration together. From our family to yours ....

May the road rise up to meet you
May the wind be always at your back
May the warm rays of sun fall upon your home
And may the hand of a friend always be near.

May green be the grass you walk on,
May blue be the skies above you,
May pure be the joys that surround you,
May true be the hearts that love you.

Irish blessing

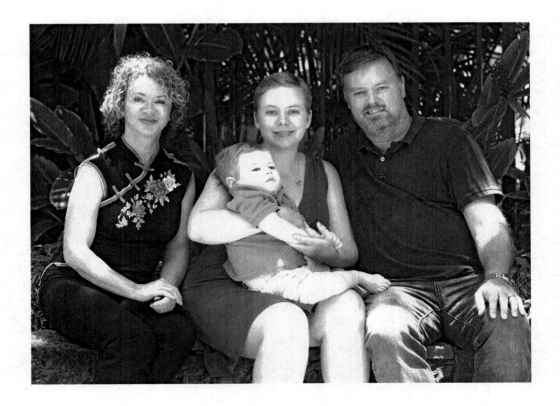

About the Authors

Aubri and Andrei Tallent and Fredy Bush started Little Bear Sees nonprofit organization in 2011 to raise awareness about cortical visual impairment (CVI) and to provide families in need with the information, products and tools to help their children with CVI learn to see. Their experience raising a child with CVI has made them particularly sensitive to the lack of knowledge that often exists among doctors, therapists and other parents. Their goal in creating the company, building www.LittleBearSees.org, developing iPad apps, and now writing this book, has been to make sure that children with CVI get the help they need so that they too can learn to see. When they are not busy advocating for children with CVI, they can often be found playing at the beach in Honolulu, Hawaii with Lukas, their Little Bear and inspiration for it all. You can contact them atcontact them at info@littlebearsees.org.

Acknowledgements

We would like to take a moment to thank the many people who have offered us their support, encouragement and knowledge on our CVI journey. We must begin by expressing our deepest gratitude to Dr. Christine Roman-Lantzy who, clearly, has informed so much of what we know about CVI. Furthermore, she gave us hope for Lukas when she mentioned the potential she saw in him. We will never forget that. We are so grateful to her for taking the time out of her incredibly busy schedule to participate in this book.

We also want to thank Kymberlee Gilkey, our amazing TVI, who opened the door that led us down this path when she first told us about cortical visual impairment. We do not want to imagine where Lukas would be today without her guidance.

In addition to Kymberlee, we must also thank everyone else on the Early Intervention team who works with Lukas and has taken the time to educate themselves about CVI. Jan Miyashiro, Liane Otake, Jihee Nguyen, Lynette Merrill, Madie Chun, Adrienne Mark, and Patricia Miko-lashek always come with smiling faces and wonderful ideas for helping Lukas. They have played no small part in the progress he has made.

Additionally, there are no words to truly express our appreciation for Lukas' physical therapist and surrogate grandmother, Jacqueline Cardoso, who offers continual love and laughter to our lives. She has helped Lukas find his strength and bolstered our own by becoming part of our family.

Our vision for this book was always to include stories from other families who have been down this path and could offer their own insights. We didn't know, at first, how many people would be willing to open up their lives and share their stories with us, and we are incredibly grateful to those who did. We offer our sincerest gratitude to the Champine family, the Williams family and the Thathachari family for taking the time to offer us all a glimpse into their world. We are so inspired by all of you.

Much of what we have been able to share with you about the role of the brain in vision has come from the work of Dr. Gordon Dutton and we are so thankful that he shared his work and expertise with us. His knowledge of the mechanics of the brain and how they are impacted by CVI has given us a much greater understanding of how to help Lukas.

Finally, this book would certainly not be what it is; in fact it would not be at all, if it weren't for the diligent, thoughtful work of Dr. Caron Goode. She conducted the interviews, did the research, and laid down the framework for our words. We simply could not have done it without her.

Resources

Parent Support Groups

Cortical Vision Impairments (groups.yahoo.com/group/Corticalvisionim-pairments), a Yahoo! support group, is dedicated to helping others understand and share ideas about cortical visual impairment and how it relates to learning.

The Jewish Guild for the Blind (www.jgb.org/programs-parent-tele.asp) offers a weekly conference call for parents of children with CVI. It is essentially a support group with guest speakers, including Dr. Roman-Lantzy, featured monthly.

Thinking Outside the Light-Box (www.facebook.com/Thinkingoutside-thelightbox) is a Facebook support group dedicated to children with CVI. It is a great place to ask questions and get ideas and suggestions from other parents.

Blogs and Websites

Babies with iPads (babieswithipads.blogspot.com) is a blog style website with reviews of apps appropriate for children with disabilities. There is a list of iPad apps (babieswithipads.blogspot.com/search?q=cvi) that they suggest are suitable for children with CVI.

FamilyConnect (www.familyconnect.org) provides videos, personal stories, events, news, and an online community that can offer tips and support from other parents of children who are blind or visually impaired.

The Independent Little Bee (adifferentkindofvision.blogspot.com) has some great information for families with visually impaired children. There are several .

Little Bear Sees (www.littlebearsees.org) is the website and blog we created to help spread the word about CVI. It includes resources, tips and facts.

SNEAK Outside the Box (www.sneakotb.com) SNEAK (Special Needs Enrichment Apps for Kids) Outside the Box is an innovative and comprehensive source for assistive technology resources to enrich the lives of children with various special needs.

Special Parent Connections (www.specialparentconnections.com) is a site where parents can read reviews on products, learn about new therapies, and find resources for themselves and their child with special needs and more. The information on this web site is based on personal experiences.

Strategy to See (www.strategytosee.com)—As a teacher of students with visual impairments, Diane Sheline developed this website, in hopes of helping parents, caretakers, teachers and all those involved with the care of children with brain damage-related vision loss, to learn methods and techniques which encourage efficient use of vision.

Wonder Baby (www.wonderbaby.org) is a great website dedicated to helping families with children who have vision impairments and multiple disabilities. They are sponsored by the Perkins School for the Blind and offer articles, reviews and a large collection of resources.

Newsletters and Journals

Council for Exceptional Children, Division on Visual Impairment Quarterly (www.cecdvi.org/DVIIQ/dviq.htm) is a newsletter with interesting ads for new products, announcements of important events, professional position papers and discussions of timely topics.

Deaf-Blind Perspectives (www.nationaldb.org/dbp) is a twice-yearly free publication on topics related to deaf-blindness. The following issue is specifically about CVI: Volume 13, Issue 3, Spring 2006, Cortical Visual Impairment: Guidelines and Educational Considerations, by Susan Edelman, Peggy Lashbrook, Annette Carey, Diane Kelly, Ruth Ann King, Christine Roman-Lantzy, and Chigee Cloniger.

Insight: Research and Practice in Visual Impairment and Blindness (www.aerbvi.org) is a new professional journal that is peer reviewed and supported by The Association for Education and Rehabilitation of the Blind and Visually Impaired (AER).

International Council for Education of People with Visual Impairment (www.icevi.org/publications)—ICEVI is the only worldwide organization supporting students with visual impairments in schools. They produce a newsletter twice a year that contains articles of interest to people in both developed and developing countries.

Journal of Blindness Innovation and Research (www.nfb-jbir.org) is another new peer reviewed journal available through the National Federation of the Blind. This journal is available online only.

The Journal of Visual Impairment and Blindness (JVIB) (www.afb.org) is often called the "journal of record" for research in this area. Articles in JVIB are peer reviewed. This journal is available in print or online in electronic format.

Continuing Education and Information

American Foundation for the Blind (www.afb.org) is another great resource for information on a variety of visual impairments. They host a comprehensive site about CVI, including some detailed articles.

American Printing House for the Blind (www.aph.org/cvi) is a great resource for information about a variety of visual impairments. They also offer a CVI information website.

The Blind Babies Foundation (www.blindbabies.org/learn/diagnoses-and-strategies) has a list of pediatric visual diagnosis fact sheets, including one about cortical visual impairment.

CONNECT (community.fpg.unc.edu/connect) is developing web-based, instructional resources for faculty and other professional development providers that focus on and respond to challenges faced each day by those working with young children with disabilities and their families. The modules help build practitioners' abilities to make evidence-based decisions.

Emerald Education Systems (www.emeraldeducationsystems.com) is an online publisher of authoritative and accredited continuing education (CE) courses with a current focus in low vision rehabilitation.

Perkins School for the Blind (www.perkins.org/resources/ask-the-expert/ellen-mazel-discusses.html) has a nice article about CVI written by Ellen Mazel, M.Ed. CTVI.

The Scottish Sensory Centre (www.ssc.education.ed.ac.uk) is funded by the Scottish Government to provide a service for Teachers of Deaf pupils, Teachers of VI pupils and Teachers of Deaf-blind pupils in Scotland, as well as other associated professionals.

Special Education Rights, Policies, and Assistance

The Council for Exceptional Children (www.cec.sped.org) is the voice and vision of special education research, accreditation and licensure information for special education teachers, administrators, and other professionals in the field.

The Early Childhood Community (community.fpg.unc.edu) is facilitated by the National Professional Development Center on Inclusion (NPDCI) and CONNECT: The Center to Mobilize Early Childhood Knowledge. It is a place to pose questions, share challenges, contribute ideas and join discussions related to the early childhood field, with an emphasis on early childhood inclusion.

Early Childhood Research and Reference Portal (www.nectac.org/portal/portal.asp) is also from NECTAC and provides links to national and state early childhood data sources, evidence-based practices, online journals, literature databases, and grants databases.

ECO (fpg.unc.edu/~eco) is the Early Childhood Outcomes Center. It provides national leadership to help states implement high-quality outcome systems for early intervention (EI) and early childhood special education (ECSE) programs.

The Families and Advocates Partnership for Education (www.fape.org) project is a partnership that aims to improve the educational outcomes for children with disabilities.

Infant and Toddlers Coordinators Association (www.ideainfanttoddler.org) is an online link to the resources that are helping to improve the lives of infants and toddlers with special needs and has interesting position papers to assist policy makers.

The National Association of Parents with Children in Special Education (www.napcse.org/exceptionalchildren/visualimpairments.php) is a national membership organization dedicated to rendering all possible support and assistance to parents whose children receive special education services, both in and outside of school. **NAPCSE** was founded for parents with children with special needs to promote a sense of community and provide a national forum for their ideas.

National Early Childhood Technical Assistance Center (www.nectac.org) is supported by the U.S. Department of Education's *Office of Special Education Programs* (OSEP) under the provisions of the Individuals with Disabilities Education Act (IDEA). The site provides a variety of resources pertaining to infant, toddler and preschool programs for children with special needs.

NICHCY, National Dissemination Center for Children with Disabilities (www.nichcy.org) is a central source of information on disabilities in infants, toddlers, children, and youth. Here, you'll also find easy-to-read information on IDEA, the law authorizing early intervention services and special education. Their will help you connect with the disability agencies and organizations in your state.

NICHCY, National Dissemination Center for Children with Disabilities, State Organization Search (www.nichcy.org/state-organization-search-by-state) allows you to search by state for organizations that can help you and your child. Every state has a Parent Training and Information Center, known as the PTI. Some states have several. If you are looking to connect with state and local resources, or have questions about services and parent rights, talk to your PTI. Find the PTI for your state by visiting the State Resource Sheets (at the address below). One of the "quick select" choices includes "Parent Training Centers."

Parent to Parent (www.p2pusa.org) provides emotional and informational support to families of children who have special needs. They can connect you with other parents like yourself, and even a trained "support parent" for support and exchange.

State eligibility definitions for infants and toddlers with disabilities under IDEA (www.nectac.org/~pdfs/pubs/nnotes21.pdf) can help you find out how your state defines developmental delay and criteria of eligibility for services to young children, birth through two years of age, and their families.

Additional Resources

The following organizations provide resources and information specifically on services for people with low vision or blindness:

American Council of the Blind
800.424.8666, info@acb.org, www.acb.org

American Foundation for the Blind
800.232.5463, afbinfo@afb.net, www.afb.org

AFB's Service Center, where you can search and identify services for blind and visually impaired persons in the United States and Canada: www.afb.org/services.asp

Blind Children's Center
www.blindchildrenscenter.org

The Foundation Fighting Blindness
(formerly the National Retinitis Pigmentosa Foundation)
800.683.5555, 800.683.5551 (TDD), info@blindness.org
www.blindness.org

Lighthouse International
800.829.0500, www.lighthouse.org

National Association for Parents of the Visually Impaired
800.562.6265, napvi@perkins.org, www.napvi.org

National Braille Association, Inc. (NBA)
www.nationalbraille.org

National Braille Press

888.965.8965, contact@nbp.org

www.nbp.org

National Eye Institute, National Institutes of Health

U.S. Department of Health and Human Services

2020@nei.nih.gov, nei.nih.gov

National Federation of the Blind

www.nfb.org/nfb

National Library Service for the Blind and Physically Handicapped

Library of Congress

888.NLS.READ, nls@loc.gov

www.loc.gov/nls

Prevent Blindness America

800.331.2020, www.preventblindness.org

Endnotes

[1] Professional interview with Dr. Christine Roman-Lantzy conducted by Dr. Caron Goode on 12-05-2011. © 2011 by Fredy Bush, Aubri Tallent and Andrei Tallent.

[2] Ibid.

[3] Ibid.

[4] Shon, K. H. "Access to the World by Visually Impaired Preschoolers." *Re:VIEW*, 30, 4 (Winter, 1999): 160-173.

[5] Schore, A. N. *Affect regulation and the origin of the self: The neurobiology of emotional development.* Hillsdale: Lawrence Erlbaum Associates, 1994.

[6] *Mayo Clinic*, http://www.mayoclinic.com/health/postpartum-depression/DS00546/DSECTION=symptoms.

[7] "What is CVI?" *American Printing House for the Blind*, http://www.aph.org/cvi/define.html.

[8] Professional interview with Dr. Christine Roman-Lantzy conducted by Dr. Caron Goode on 12-05-2011. © 2011 by Fredy Bush, Aubri Tallent and Andrei Tallent.

[9] Ibid.

[10] California Deaf Blind Services. "Neurological Visual Impairment: Also Known as Cortical Visual Impairment, Delayed Visual Maturation, Cortical Blindness." Found at *American Printing House for the Blind*, http://www.aph.org/cvi/articles/cdbs_1.html.

[11] Good, W.V., James E Jan, Susan K Burden, Ann Skoczenski, and Rowan Candy. "Recent advances in cortical visual impairment." *American Printing House for the Blind,* http://www.aph.org/cvi/articles/good_1.html.

[12] Groenveld, M. "Children with Cortical Visual Impairment." *American Printing House for the Blind,* http://www.aph.org/cvi/articles/groenveld_1.html.

[13] K. Appleby's compiling information from article by: Jan, J.E., A. Groen-veld, A.M. Sykanda, and C.S. Hoyt. "Behavioral Characteristics of Children with Permanent Cortical Visual Impairment." *Developmental Medicine & Child Neurology*, 25 (1987): 755-762. Information provided by Vision Associates, 2109 US Hwy 90 West, Ste. 170 #312, Lake City, FL 32055.

[14] Harrell, L. "Cortical Visual Impairment – A Challenging Diagnosis." *American Printing House for the Blind*, http://www.aph.org/cvi/articles/harrell_1.html.

[15] Shatz, C.J. "Emergence of order in visual system development." *Journal of Physiology-Paris* 90, 3-4, (1996): 141-150.

[16] Boothe R.G., V. Dobson, and D.Y. Teller. "Postnatal development of vision in human and nonhuman primates." *Annual Review of Neuroscience* 8 (1985):495.

[17] "Infant Vision: Birth to 24 Months of Age." *American Optometric Association*, http://www.aoa.org/x9420.xml#1.

[18] Rybak, I.A. "A model of attention-guided visual perception and recognition." *Vision Research* 38 (1998): 2387–2400.

[19] Good, W.V., James E Jan, Susan K Burden, Ann Skoczenski, Rowan Candy. "Recent advances in cortical visual impairment." *American Printing House for the Blind,* http://www.aph.org/cvi/articles/good_1.html.

[20] Hoyt, C. S. "Visual function in the brain-damaged child." *Eye* 17 (2003): 369-384.

[21] Dutton, G.N. "Visual problems in children with damage to the brain." *American Printing House for the Blind,* http://www.aph.org/cvi/articles/dutton_1.html.

[22] Good, W. V., J.E. Jan, L. DeSa, A.J. Barkovich, M. Groenveld, and C.S. Hoyt. "Cortical visual impairment in children." *Survey of Ophthalmology 38*, 4 (1994): 351-364.

[23] Baker-Nobles, L. and A. Rutherford. "Understanding cortical visual

impairment in children." *The American Journal of Occupational Therapy* 49, 9 (1995): 899-903.

[24] Roman-Lantzy, C. *Cortical Visual Impairment: An Approach to Assessment and Intervention.* New York City: American Foundation for the Blind Press, 2007. p. 23.

[25] Jan, J. E., and P. K. H. Wong. "The child with cortical visual impairment." *Seminars in Ophthalmology* 6, 4 (1991): 194-200.

[26] "Description of Light Box – Revised!" *American Printing House for the Blind,* https://shop.aph.org/webapp/wcs/stores/servlet/ProductDisplay?storeId= 10001&catalogId=11051&krypto=w%2FE%2FZ6s4BbOTWTAk7uwYkwPqZ0g DTT8mPqLLyhhVaTsq5cuSkOiPy5BjiL90i%2FEyDtBzvF%2FUJVgS%0D%0A5f zQRbG3dg%3D%3D&ddkey=http:ProductDisplay (accessed by Dr. Caron Goode on 03-15-12).

[27] Blind Babies Foundation. "Cortical Visual Impairment Pediatric Visual Diagnosis Fact Sheet." *American Printing House for the Blind,* http://www.aph.org/cvi/articles/bbf_1.html.

[28] Faverjon, S., D. C. Silveira, D. D. Fu, B. H. Cha, C. Akman, Y. Hu and G. L. Holmes. "Beneficial effects of enriched environment following status epilepticus in immature rats." *Neurology* 59, 9 (Nov 12, 2002): 1356-1364.

[29] Ibid.

[30] Gravel, M., Y.C. Weng, and J. Kriz. "Model system for living imaging of neuronal responses to injury and repair." *Molecular Imaging* 10, 6 (Dec 1, 2011): 434-45.

[31] Buonomano D.V. and M.M. Merzenich. "Cortical plasticity: from synapses to maps." *Annual Review of Neuroscience* 21 (1998):149-86.

[32] Kempermann G., E.P. Brandon, and F.H. Gage. "Environmental stimulation of 129/Svj mice causes increased cell proliferation and neurogenesis in the adult dentate gyrus." *Current Biology* 8 (1998): 939-942.

[33] Amen, D. *Change Your Brain, Change Your Life*. New York: Three Rivers Press, 1998.

[34] Doidge, N. *The Brain That Changes Itself*. New York: Penguin, 2007.

[35] Roman-Lantzy, C. *Cortical Visual Impairment: An Approach to Assessment and Intervention*. New York City: American Foundation for the Blind Press, 2007.

[36] Professional interview with Dr. Christine Roman-Lantzy conducted by Dr. Caron Goode on 12-05-2011. © 2011 by Fredy Bush, Aubri Tallent and Andrei Tallent.

[37] Lantzy, C.A.R and A. Lantzy. "Outcomes and Opportunities: A Study of Children with Cortical Visual Impairment." *Journal of Visual Impairment and Blindness* 104, 10 (October 2010): 649-653.

[38] McDaid, G., Debbie Cockburn, Gordon N Dutton. "Devising strategies to optimise home and school life for children with visual impairment due to damage to the brain." *Scottish Sensory Centre*, http://www.ssc.education.ed.ac.uk/courses/vi&multi/vjan08ii.html.

[39] Unsicker, C. "Winning Strategies for Lowest Functioning CVI Students." Presentation CTEBVI Workshop, #805, Oakland, CA. (March 12, 2011).

[40] "Ketogenic Diet." *Epilepsy Foundation*, http://www.epilepsyfoundation.org/aboutepilepsy/treatment/keto-genicdiet/index.cfm?gclid=CMbltfiq6q4CFQIvhwodYlYDLg.

[41] Dutton, G.N. "Cerebral Visual Impairment: Working Within and Around the Limitations of Vision." In *Proceedings of the Summit on Cerebral/Cortical Visual Impairment: Educational, Family, and Medical Perspectives*, edited by E. Dennison and A. Hall Lueck, 3-26. New York: American Foundation for the Blind Press, 2006.

[42] "Overview of Early Intervention." *NICHCY*, http://nichcy.org/babies/overview#included.

[43] "Supports, Modifications and Accommodations for Students." *NICHCY*, http://nichcy.org/schoolage/accommodations/.

[44] Ibid.

[45] Murphy, R. "Learning-Related Vision Problems." *All About Vision*, http://www.allaboutvision.com/parents/learning.htm.